Massage for
Total Well-Being

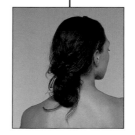

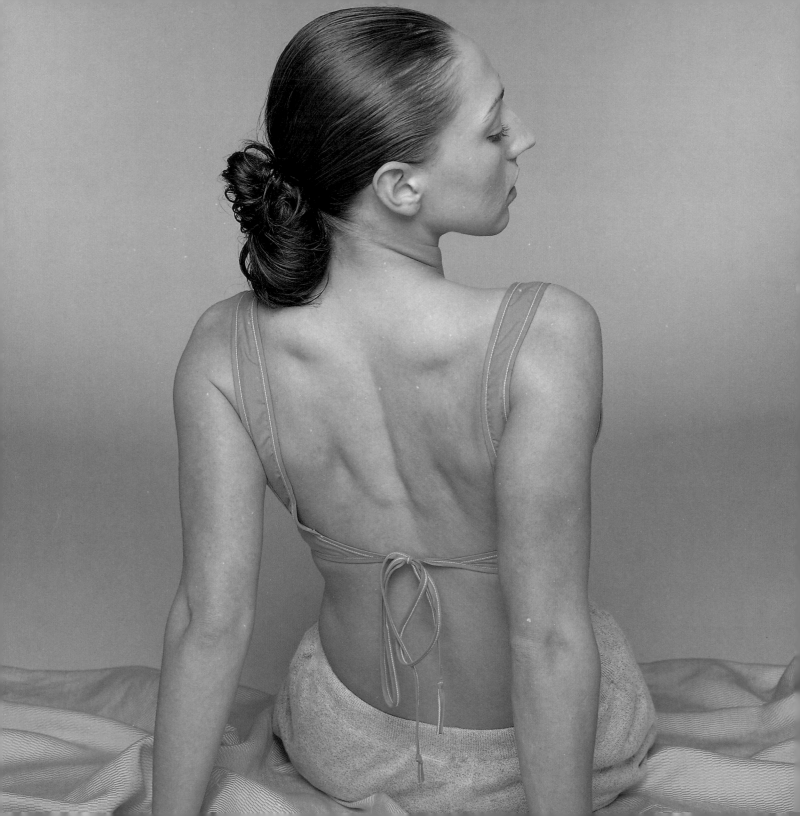

Massage for Total Well-Being

*Massage and Meditation
for the Seven Centers of Health*

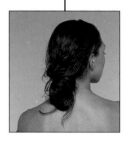

Anne Kent Rush

Photographs by Victoria Rauhofer

A Byron Preiss Book
UNIVERSE

First published in the United States of America in 2000
by UNIVERSE PUBLISHING
A Division of Rizzoli International Publications, Inc.
300 Park Avenue South
New York, NY 10010

2000 2001 2002 2003 2004 2005 / 10 9 8 7 6 5 4 3 2 1

Printed in Singapore

Designed by Karen Healy
Storyboard for illustrations by Anne Kent Rush

Library of Congress Cataloging-in-Publication Data

Rush, Anne Kent, 1945-
    Massage for total well-being : massage and meditation for the seven centers of health /
Anne Kent Rush ; photographs by Victoria Rauhofer.
        p. cm.
    "A Byron Preiss book."
    Includes bibliographical references
    ISBN 0-7893-0490-2 (hardcover)
    1. Massage. I. Title.

RA780.5 .R8725 2000
615.8'22--dc21

                                                                00-055944

Massage for
Total Well-Being

Contents

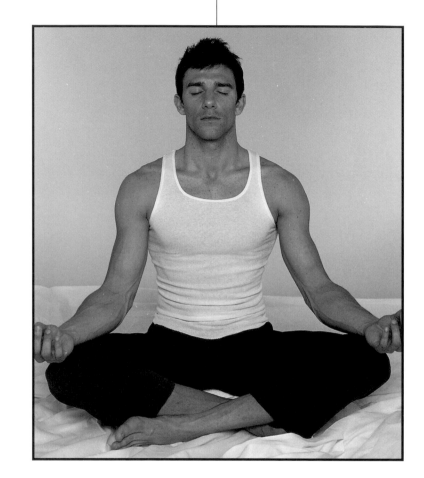

Section | Two

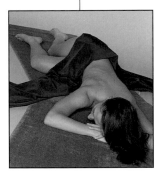

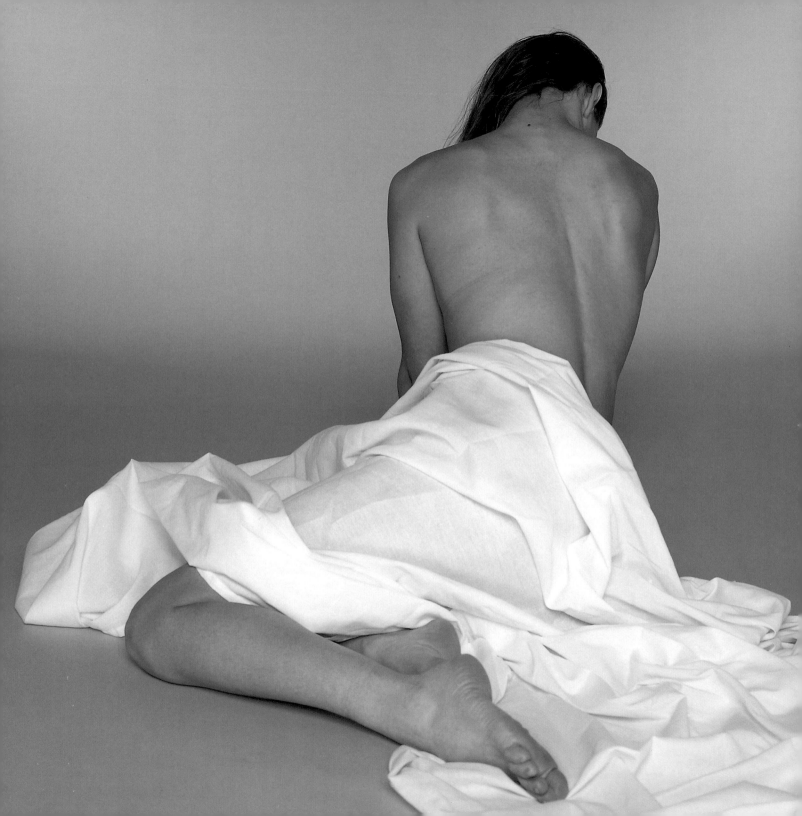

Introduction

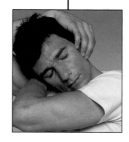

Agood massage involves our total being—touch, smell, sound, emotions, nerves, mind, muscle, and spirit. The closer we look at our bodies with the aid of science and technology, the less substantial and more mysterious they become. Growing numbers of respected health professionals agree with medical doctor Deepak Chopra, who writes, "The three-dimensional body reported by the five senses is a mirage. . . . Beyond the quantum, your body exists as pure creative potential, a multilayered process controlled by intelligence." Incorporating this concept of ourselves as evolving communities of cells into our practical lives is the health challenge of the new millennium. How can we put this idea into practice? If we are fluid beings, composed of interrelated and evolving parts, how can we massage that?

Happily, discovering the answer means our lives can have more depth and pleasure. It means bringing relaxation and balance into all aspects of our lives. Since body and mind are one, to produce your best mental work at the office, you need to be physically comfortable and sensually stimulated. The office chair needs to be tailor-fitted for your health. To revive your senses, your work space could include a photograph of a beautiful scene in nature or a vase of your favorite flowers. Periods of mental stress should be balanced by physical treats such as a walk or a massage.

One of the best methods for total revival of body and spirit is massage. Few easily accessible treatments can renew a person so completely. Dr. Candace Pert, the remarkable neuroscientist who discovered our bodies' opiate receptors, counsels, "Feeling anxious, worthless? Get a massage. . . . Your mind, your feelings are in your body, and it's there, in your somatic experience, that feeling is healed."

In this newest of new ages, we look for more out of an exercise or a spa treatment than simply improving the shapes of our bodies. Dr. Caroline Myss, the pioneer in energy medicine, asserts, "healing begins with the repair of emotional injuries. Our entire medical model is being reshaped around the power of the heart." We understand the need to address our total being, to focus our minds and soothe our spirits as well. By incorporating aromatherapy, kinesthesiology, and meditation, massage now includes healing for all the senses. While massage and health spas are traditions thousands of years old, it may have taken us all these years to fully embrace the power and the possibilities of ancient hands-on treatments, and to learn to use them in our plan for total health. Yet, touch has always been at the core of good health care, and its most popular form is massage.

Hands-on Health

Gentle touch is healing—we know this by instinct and by experience. In the twenty-first century, science is making headway with new technology that is able to test and prove what common sense has told us before. Dr. Christiane Northrup writes in *Women's Bodies, Women's Wisdom*: "We must begin to trust ourselves and our experience as much as we trust laboratory data." Today many insurance policies accept massage as treatment for injuries, and many doctors prescribe it for reducing stress and for intensifying the powers of other medical remedies.

As the pace of our lives accelerates, as change and shock increase in our everyday experience, and as medical costs continue to rise, we need more than ever to learn to take better care of our own health and of those we love. Massage is always relaxing, sometimes deeply healing, and usually easily available to us all. Besides, it's fun. What else that's so good for us is so pleasurable?

The earliest written record of massage, named from an Arabic word meaning *stroke*, appeared three thousand years ago in China, and the Chinese health system has retained an uninterrupted knowledge and respect for its healing power. The fourth-century Greek father of modern Western medicine, Hippocrates, insisted that his physicians be expert masseurs. Only fairly recently in history has massage been considered suspect. In the Middle Ages, the church proclaimed manipulation of the body the work of the devil. In August 1997, *Life* magazine reported, "In the twentieth century, massage has often been assumed to be a front—not for the devil but for prostitution." While studying massage in Berkeley in 1970, in the hope that the twenty-first century would be different, I decided to do my part to remedy this unfortunate misconception.

As of 1970, medical texts provided the only information on massage, and the techniques were known only by medical practitioners and the occasional pro-sports trainer. As both a massage enthusiast and a writer, I was inspired to produce a massage manual for the layperson. I thought, "Shouldn't everyone have these healing processes available to them and their families?"

In 1971 I began teaching at the Esalen Institute in California and worked often with George Downing, a therapist. I lead training groups for health professionals on how to integrate body-therapy techniques into traditional medical practice. I suggested my idea to George and he agreed to write the text; I would edit and illustrate it. Don Gerrard, managing editor of the Bookworks, was adventurous enough to take on the project when nobody else thought the general public would be interested, and we co-published *The Massage Book* with Random House in 1971. The book caught on like wildfire and is still in print today, enjoying an exceptional publishing life. Having been a part of bringing massage into modern American living gives me great satisfaction.

In health clubs, rehab clinics, resort spas, baby as well as geriatric treatments, family homes, and romantic hideaways, it's nearly impossible to imagine life in the United States today without massage. Increasingly, American medical doctors are tapping the resources of massage for their work. The Touch Research Institute in Miami has provided valuable scientific data on the medically healing effects of massage. Their work in improving the health of premature babies with massage is particularly impressive and has clear implications for treatment of people of all ages. The babies at TRI receive three massages a day for ten days. The result is that the babies are more alert, active, and responsive than nonmassaged infants. The babies also sleep more deeply, tolerate noise better, gain weight 47 percent faster, have fewer episodes of breath cessation (apnea), and leave the hospital six days sooner than nonmassaged babies. In other cases, gentle touch can be the difference between life and death, offering a person relief from suffering and the promise of improvement that instigates the will to live. Massage reminds us that life can be good.

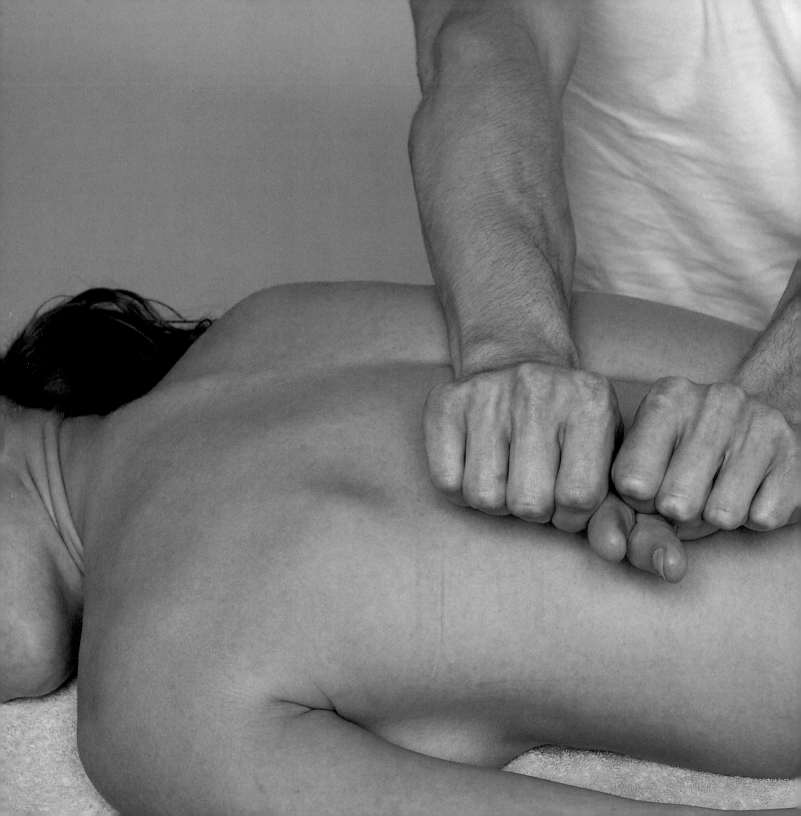

Total
Well-Being

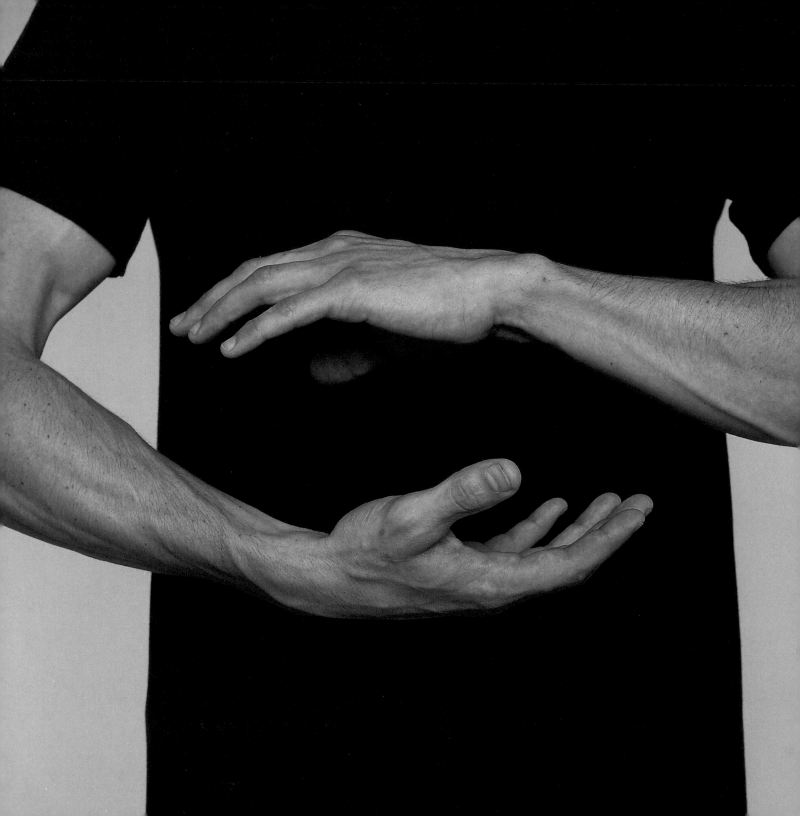

The Well-Being Spa

The Future of Self-Care

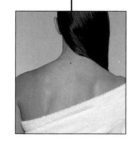

Aspa is a place to go to revive oneself from stress and to form new habits that will enrich our bodies and spirits. To embrace Drs. Chopra, Myss, and Pert's new paradigm that healing requires both mind and body, each topic in this book is formed in paired sections of a spirit spa with meditation and a body spa with massage. The individual treatments are also tailor-made to express this new understanding. Each massage focuses on body areas corresponding to one of the seven key energy centers delineated in most major spiritual belief systems. I have chosen to use the energy terminology from Hindu yoga because it is more familiar to many yoga-practicing Westerners, including myself, than the related, but more esoteric, Buddhist, Christian, or Judaic systems. Yet, all the energy systems are remarkably similar. As Dr. Caroline Myss writes in her book *Anatomy of the Spirit*, "Within the four major religions is the [concept] that the divine is locked into our biological system in seven stages of power that lead us to become more refined and transcendent in our personal power."

If you have been practicing or receiving massage for quite a while, you may be in transition about how to work according to the new health model. If you are new to the world of massage, you have a chance to form your habits based on an understanding of the body that includes all aspects of a person, and at a time when the Western medical community recognizes massage's health benefits more than ever.

The basic massages are presented for each of the seven energy centers to demonstrate how to practice based on this mind/body paradigm. People involved in bodywork often experience connections between mind and body. Massage can elicit a memory or emotion triggered by touch to a specific area. Most massage therapists encourage the exploration of those feelings by talking about them or by visualizing their sequence with a variety of conclusions to offer resolution options. Today, because of advanced equipment, we have scientific explanations for how emotions are stored in various body areas and about the chemistry of their functioning. The most accessible scientific resource is Dr. Candace Pert's *Molecules of Emotion*. Also, we now have the thorough fieldwork of Dr. Myss, reported in *Anatomy of the Spirit*, outlining a precise model for working with psychological connections between body parts and emotions, and between physical ailments and mental states. *Massage for Total Well-Being* adds to this area by applying these concepts to the practice of massage and by combining your massage with meditation to deepen and balance the experience.

Relaxation Is More than Skin Deep

Massage complemented by meditation can become the core of a comprehensive health and stress-management regimen. Modern research shows that massage, no longer an expensive splurge on special occasions, should become part of our health routine, much like getting a haircut or flossing our teeth but with broader, more profound benefits. By incorporating the techniques from this book into your daily routine, you will create a healthier and more pleasurable future for your body and mind because of the prolonged physiological and psychological benefits of massage and meditation.

In modern society, our body's natural rhythms often become thwarted by the rapid momentum of technology, causing stress, pain, and illness. Ask anyone today, "How do you feel?" and their response will usually be, "Tense," "tired," "anxious," "in pain." These by-products of our lifestyle have become so pervasive, most of us assume these stressed states are normal and continuous. We forget what it feels like to feel good, to feel healthy, to function in sync with our natural rhythms.

Recent medical studies of stress-related illnesses point to the necessity of positive physical contact for human health. Studies show that blocked emotions can be released through forms of deep massage, proving that touch not only builds muscle tone and improves circulation but also dissolves unhealthy defenses. A recent medical study from the University of California at Berkeley has found that to break a bad habit one must not only eliminate the negative action, one must also substitute a positive one for it if the change is to last. This indicates that massage could be effective in the treatment of addiction.

A massage feels so good that most people need little urging to indulge. But few people know of the specific medical and psychological effects. At the Touch Research Institute, psychologist Tiffany Field heads a staff of therapists and students who collaborate with researchers at Duke, the University of Miami, and Harvard. They have discovered that massage reduces agitation in Alzheimer's patients, improves health in premature babies, helps asthmatics breathe better, boosts immune function in HIV-positive patients, improves students' ability to concentrate, lowers anxiety in the depressed, and reduces fear in trauma patients. C. Gillon Ward, the medical director of Jackson's Burn Center, says, "I started out thinking it was a bunch of hooey, but I've become a believer."

Psychiatrist James Gordon states, "Massage is medicine." We know instinctively that an encouraging touch can mean the difference between giving up and going on when words may fail. Our skin holds as many as five million touch receptors. There are three thousand in one fingertip. They are there for a purpose—actually, a multitude of purposes. Each touch receptor's nerve sends messages along the spinal cord to the brain. These messages vary from reducing heart rate to increasing natural opiates to improving food absorption and muscle coordination.

There are sometimes long-term results that come from regular massages. But the immediate results of loving touch are just as extraordinary as the long-term ones—we feel happier. We experience a sense of connectedness with others. We are renewed by a pat on the back or a gentle stroke on the cheek. Through learning more about the wide variety of massage techniques, we are really learning how to communicate better. With the spas in this book we can improve and expand the ways we touch each other, physically and spiritually, throughout our lives.

The Seven Chakras of the Body

The Spirit Spa

Energy at the Gym

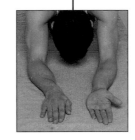

At health spas today, there is a heartening movement away from superficial pampering and toward more in-depth explorations of paths to inner beauty. Meditation in many forms often accompanies massage in a move toward balancing inner and outer serenity.

Our energy systems need stretching as much as our muscles do. Most of us would like to be able to increase or calm our energy levels at will. Western medicine and athletic systems offer a variety of drugs and techniques aimed at energy control. Asian disciplines can add valuable information to Western efforts because they offer detailed maps of the body's energy systems plus many natural, nondrug techniques for energy management.

In Indian medical and spiritual terminology, energy (*prana*) is believed to come from the air. "Most of the energy for the body we get from the air we breathe, and not, as is commonly assumed, from food and water," writes Swami Vishnudevananda in *The Complete Illustrated Book of Yoga*. Traditional Japanese medicine, philosophy, and martial arts name the life energy *ki*. Chinese medicine and spiritual practices call life energy *ch'i*.

In Chinese medicine, appropriate energy flow through the body is considered the most important indicator and source of good health. "Energy imbalance—its excess or insufficiency—is the root of illness, its absence is death," writes Dr. Yoshio Manaka in *The Layman's Guide to Acupuncture*.

Acupuncture, a traditional Chinese medical system, was developed more than four thousand years ago. Medical practitioners observed that specific places on the body are sensitive or sore on an ailing person. A chart of these places defines lines, or meridians, connecting the points that affect one another most directly. Western science acknowledges and has measured the existence in the body of such meridians, or electromagnetic currents, that can affect health. The Chinese names for the negative and positive charges of body electricity are *yin* and *yang*. Imbalance of these two currents in our bodies is seen as the root of all health problems.

> *Rosemary and lemon scents piped into Japanese office buildings increase worker productivity.*

Western doctors use "electrostim" treatments and physical therapy to revive damaged muscles. Asian medicine uses acupuncture and exercise. *The Layman's Guide to Acupuncture* is a helpful book for practical use. As you massage a body part, you stimulate the energy center located there. When you stimulate your skin and muscles, you are also balancing and recharging your whole electrical energy system.

Body/Mind Energy Centers

In Indian yoga terminology, a biological nerve plexus, or center, is called a *chakra*, a junction for spiritual as well as physical energy. Western science recognizes biological nerve centers in these areas. Eastern understanding of the body adds a mental and emotional dominant characteristic to each nerve center. Medical pioneers such as Drs. Myss, Chopra, and Pert have discovered the validity of this thinking about how the body really functions. This knowledge is useful when we focus on health. Balancing the mental qualities tied to a physical part produces a more effective treatment or massage. The exercises in this book offer relaxation for both aspects.

The Seven Chakras

Pelvic Plexus: Kundalini chakra—sex organs; starting point of the body's life-energy flow at the base of the spine; basic molecular health and balance. Associated with relationship to the earth, basic security, and family.

Belly Plexus: Navel chakra—abdomen; center of physical and spiritual balance; sense of self and inner calm; creativity and control.

Solar Plexus: Diaphragm chakra—rib cage area; channel for outer-directed power; sense of self-esteem and responsibility; trust and values.

Cardiac Plexus: Heart chakra—center of love and compassion; can infuse all other chakras with these qualities. Related to heart, circulatory system, and thymus gland.

Throat Plexus: Throat chakra—cervical ganglion, thyroid gland, parathyroid, vagus nerve, mouth, neck. Associated with willpower, creative capacity, judgment, and communication.

Forehead Plexus: Mental chakra—"Third Eye" pineal gland; intuition; center of clear, rational perception; honest vision of self and others.

Cranial Plexus: Spiritual chakra—pituitary gland; top of head. Associated with sense of perspective and unity with other forms of life; faith, selflessness, and ethics. Related to skull and skeletal system, as well as general energy in body.

Aromatherapy

That certain scents help heal specific medical problems is a concept thousands of years old. Generally it is the essential oil of a plant that imparts the scent. When a plant that contains natural essential oil is touched, squeezed, or peeled, tiny drops of oil mist into the air and fill our noses with the plant's characteristic aroma. Essential oils are usually available at health food stores or natural cosmetics stores. Extracting essential oils to preserve their aromatic essences is an art. Synthetic scents have little of the healing qualities that natural scents do. To enjoy the benefits of aromatherapy you can purchase incense with your chosen scent. Or you may mix your own meditation scents and massage oils from essential oils.

Stress Management

Relatively minor yet frequent annoyances have a more destructive effect on our health than do grand-scale traumas. This was the conclusion of a study on stress conducted by Richard Lazarus and his colleagues at the University of California, Berkeley. With stress, it's the little things that mean a lot.

The good news is that small tension-relief sessions performed frequently throughout the day can have a big effect on relieving stress. Make healing a way of life. Include short stretching and breathing breaks in each day's routine to keep the little stresses from snowballing. Take a moment to bend over in your chair and relax your back several times a day. Sprinkle brief exercises or self-administered pressure point massage revivers throughout your daily routine. You'll be doing yourself a big preventive favor.

Full Rest

Resting should be so simple. However, sometimes we're too tense to relax. If so, the following gentle sequence can make you aware of your anxieties and muscle cramps so you can release them gradually. Practiced over time, it can help you sleep more soundly.

1 Lie down on your back on a flat surface with your arms resting at your sides and your palms up. Clear your mind of all thoughts other than the feelings in your body. Make a mental note of how your body feels lying on the floor. Starting with your feet, notice which parts of your body touch the floor and which parts arch away. Do you feel tilted in any direction?

2 Flex and release each joint and muscle, working up to the head. Inhale as you flex; exhale as you release. Imagine that your breathing can massage you from the inside, as though you could exhale through your body and into any tight areas to soften them. Try visualizing that you are resting on a soft, green bed of clover in a sunny field.

3 When you reach your head, compare how your body feels now to when you started. This exercise, practiced over time, will train you to release muscle tension and to feel more "at home" and secure in your body.

Breath Spa

> *Even more than getting massages, giving them lowers stress hormones and calms the giver to a measurable physiological degree.*

At the core of body rhythm, the breath is like a snowflake, displaying a unique natural pattern in each person. An individual's rhythm can provoke strong reactions in others. You can be drawn to or antagonized by someone because he or she is speedy or slow-paced, unpredictable or consistent. Learning to recognize your own rhythm can broaden insight into your moods, offer you more control over your physical states, improve your ability to minimize stress, and raise your athletic performance.

When active, you breathe relatively quickly and high in your chest. Holding the breath is a sign of tense anticipation. Slow breathing is a sign of relaxation and repose. Deep breathing is a partner of deep emotion. Most of the time our breathing rhythms occur unconsciously, without our noticing them or how much they affect our moods.

If you consciously change your breathing rhythm, you'll find this alters your emotional state. Breath control is a useful relaxation skill in any situation, one that needs no equipment, privacy, or extra time.

The volume of our daily intake of air is five times greater than our daily intake of fluid and food. The lungs need exercise to function well, just as joints and muscles do.

Healthy movement and exercise require that sufficient oxygen reach our muscles. Deep breathing increases the flow. Because we need to clear our lungs of stale air to make space for fresh air, it is key to exhale fully. In general, do not hold your breath during exertion. Inhale as you stretch out; exhale as you bend or pull in. Synchronize your motion with your breathing. Inhale as you extend or lift. Exhale as you release or bend. The major release of tension occurs on the exhalation, as your muscles "let go."

You need to learn to find the natural breathing rhythm you would have if no outside influences interfered. This rhythm can be found using the Basic Breath exercise. Once you have a sense of your own relaxed rhythm, you have a middle point from which to gauge variations in a spectrum from very tense to very relaxed. Anytime you want to relax, it's simple to do the Basic Breath and improve your state.

The Basic Breath can be used for healing—to increase circulation in an area, to speed up tissue regeneration after injury, to relieve the pain of headaches and backaches, and to help you sleep. It also can be used to dramatically improve your physical agility and coordination by giving you a sensitivity to and control over your body rhythms.

The Basic Breath: Find Yourself While Floating on Air

The Basic Breath exercise was developed by Magdalene Proskauer, a San Francisco therapist. This breathing cycle is designed to trigger your natural rhythm gradually. By using this cycle you can let go of imposed rhythms and allow your own rhythm to surface. Find yourself while floating on air.

1 Lie on your back on the bed or floor. Relax your arms at your sides and let your feet fall out to the sides. Close your eyes and feel the way you are lying. Notice whether any part of your body feels a bit tense or doesn't seem to be resting comfortably on the surface beneath you. Now move your focus inside your body and notice where you feel movement as you breathe.

2 If you feel tense anywhere, try imagining that you can breathe into the tension, as though you could actually exhale through that body part. Imagine the breath relaxing your sore muscles as it moves through them. Breathing into a body part is something you can do anywhere, anytime you feel tense or nervous. Locate the tight place and "breathe into it." Breathe in sync with the tensing (inhale) and relaxing (exhale) of your movement.

3 As you are doing this exercise, loosen your clothing if it is binding. Let the muscles of your stomach and abdomen relax, and let your breath sink lower in your body. Place one palm down at the lowest part on your torso where you can feel the motion of your breathing. Let your hand rest on this place until you begin to feel the rise and fall of your body under your palm from your breathing. Now let your hand and arm relax at your side again. If you see any pictures of yourself or other images during this breathing exercise, remember them and draw or write them down later. They are waking dreams and can be clues to your deeper feelings about yourself and your environment. You can interpret them as you would your other dreams.

4 Relax your jaw and open your mouth a little so that you can exhale through your mouth. You don't need to breathe heavily. Relax and breathe naturally. Inhale through your nose, exhale through your mouth, and pause at the end of the exhalation before you breathe again.

The Pause

The pause is the key to the effectiveness of the breathing exercises. Crucial things are happening to your body during the pause; you are actually still exhaling, though you may feel as though nothing is going on. Deepening your exhalation gets all the stale air out of your lungs and makes more room for fresh air when you inhale. Most of us don't exhale deeply enough. Often, when you feel that you can't take in enough air and that you'd like to inhale more deeply, it's because you haven't exhaled fully enough to make room in your lungs for new air. This is usually the breathing difficulty in asthma. Lengthening your exhalation can help relieve asthmatic symptoms.

You have paused at the end of the exhalation for a long time now. Let yourself really explore the pause. How does it feel to you? Does it feel too long? Not long enough? Are you a little worried that your body won't breathe in again unless you make it? Think of animals breathing when they are resting. Their breath is long and rolling. They don't tell themselves to breathe. You can learn to trust that your breath will always come in again.

Allow the pause to be as long as it wants. It may feel very long. See whether you can wait and stay with the pause until your body wants to breathe in again by itself. Inhale through your nose, exhale through your mouth, then pause and wait. It's a little like standing on the beach and waiting for another wave to come in. Try to find a pace at which you are neither holding your breath to prolong the pause nor making yourself breathe in again. Let yourself breathe in this pattern as long as you want.

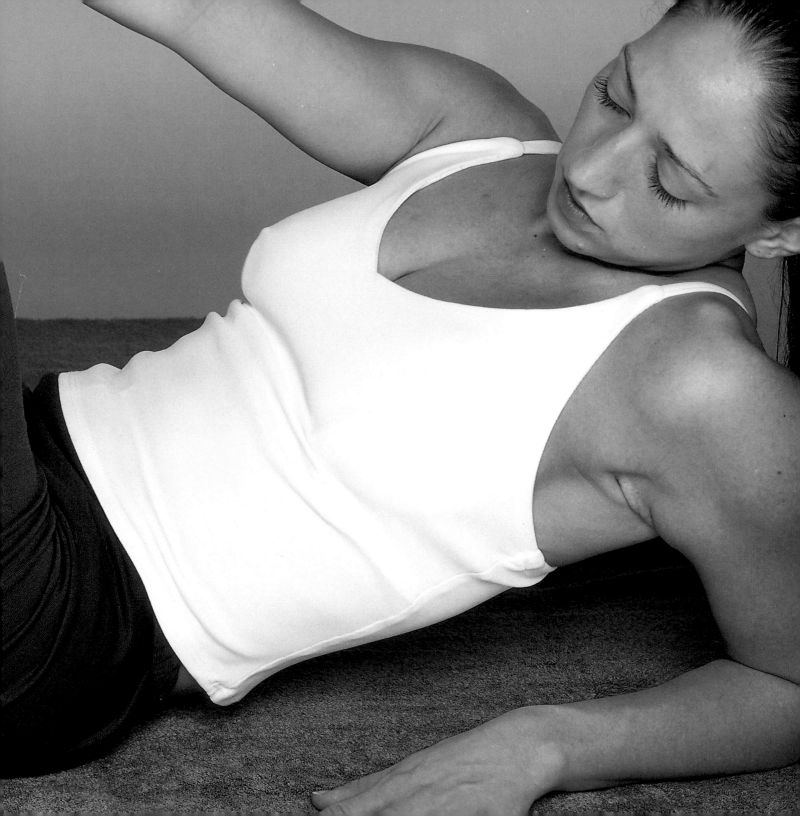

The Pause exercise in itself is deeply relaxing. If you have difficulty going to sleep, you can use this breath at night. Or, anytime you feel tense, you can take a few minutes off for yourself, relax, and find your rhythm again.

Breathing Energy

You can apply the Basic Breath to your exercises, to massage, and even to pain relief. By imagining you are breathing into a body part, you stimulate circulation in that area. More blood flows to the painful spot, warming it, bringing more oxygen to decrease aching, carrying away waste materials from the cells, and generally reviving and relaxing the tissue. What you usually sense as a result of breathing into the body part is a warming and softening of the muscle and sometimes a tingling sensation from the change in circulation. This relaxation of the tissue will immediately cause some relief of your aches and pains. For relief of severe pain, continue the breathing process longer. No body part is unreachable by the breath.

Adding a small movement to your breathing exercise can also increase its effectiveness at relieving pain. Although you need not be in any particular position, the quickest pain relief comes from doing the exercise while lying down flat or with knees bent, because you can give over the work of holding up your weight to the bed or floor and put all your attention on relaxing. Synchronize the motions with your breathing. Inhale as you lift or stretch. Exhale as you release or bend. To use the Basic Breath if you are giving a massage, imagine you can exhale down your arms, into your hands, and send warm energy into your friend's body. When you are receiving a massage, use the Pause exercise, and imagine you can direct your breathing into whatever body part is being massaged.

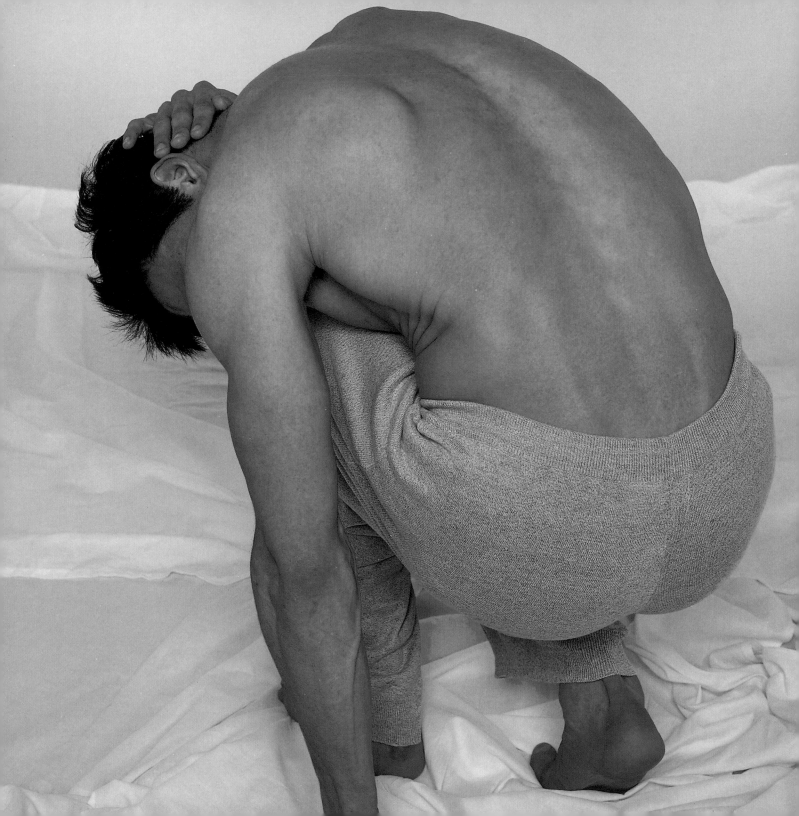

The Body Spa

Massage Preparation

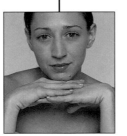

When planning to give a massage to a friend, there are several things you should do to prepare. Choose a quiet room. Use a beach towel over a soft or smooth surface, such as a rug, or a massage table with a foam pad. Talk as little as possible—this time is for body language.

If you are standing to give the massage, keep your feet about shoulder-width apart and bend your knees slightly at all times. Have a squeeze bottle of warm massage oil within easy reach. As you bend over for deep strokes, let the weight of your leaning body supply most of the pressure, rather than trying to exert pressure by pushing with your arms. Keeping these tips in mind will prevent strain on your own back as you massage, and your partner will appreciate the increased strength and ease of your motion. Always spread enough oil on the area to be massaged so your hands will glide with little friction over the skin.

In a study of casual touch between couples in cafes around the world, most cultures rated between 70 and 180 times per hour; the United States rate was lowest, at 2 times per hour.

Although two-person massage can be deeply relaxing, you may need a pick-me-up when no outside help is in sight. A great number of the massage strokes can be done on yourself. These are indicated in the text by an asterisk next to the stroke title.

Centering: A Good Way to Begin and End

Have your friend lie down and close his or her eyes. Rest the palms of your hands on the shoulders to make light physical contact before the massage strokes begin. Take a few moments to close your eyes, relax your breathing, and focus your own energy. As you massage, try to synchronize your strokes with your breathing rhythm. This will add a deeper sense of relaxation to the whole experience. You'll always want your right hand (positive charge) on the abdomen or lower back and your left hand (negative charge) toward the top of the body to maintain energy flow from the base of the spine upward.

Here are a few soothing positions.

- If your friend is lying on his or her back, stand to the right. Rest your left palm on the top of the head and your right palm below the navel on the abdomen.

- If your friend is lying on his or her stomach, stand to the left. Rest your left palm on the top of the head (or the top of the back), and rest your right palm on the sacrum bone at the base of the spine.

- Rest with your palms on both of your friend's feet.

- Rest both your palms on your friend's upturned palms.

- When you are ready to end the massage, pause for several seconds of centering again to wrap the experience in moments of gentle stillness. Always release hand contact slowly. Allow your friend to rest on the table as long as he or she wants before rising.

Palm Power*

This exercise will heighten the power of your massage. For centuries, martial-arts masters, healers, and yogis felt subtle currents during their practice and included systems for directing the currents to deepen the energizing effects of their movements and to heal strains and pains. Modern scientific equipment now exists that can locate and measure electromagnetic currents in the body. You can do a simple exercise with your hands to feel these currents. The experience offers you a way to extend the range of your movements and send energy all over your body. Initially try this technique with your hands. Later you can try directing the energy to any part of your (or someone else's) body during massage to increase relaxation and healing.

1 Sit comfortably, eyes closed, hands resting palms up on your knees. Relax any tense muscles you feel by imagining that each time you exhale, a little more tension leaves your body. Allow your breathing to sink low in your body so that your belly puffs out a bit as you inhale and sinks back in as you exhale.

2 Now imagine what it would feel like if you could send your exhalation through the center of your body, through your torso, to massage your muscles from the inside. Allow your breath to bring warmth and air to any tight areas. As you breathe, oxygen is drawn into your body and spreads to various parts through your bloodstream.

3 As you exhale, imagine you can send air down through your shoulders and arms and eventually into your hands. What would it feel like if you could exhale down your arms and out the center of your palms, through a spot about the size of a quarter?

4 Raise your palms so they are facing each other at about waist height. The increased circulation to your hands as a result of your breathing sometimes brings a sense of warmth and tingling. The muscle relaxation and improved circulation allow the body's electric currents to move more easily. Can you feel any sense of this electric flow between your facing palms?

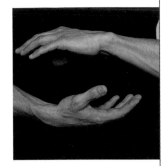

Some positions intensify the current flow. Allow your hands to move slowly in any direction they want. Try holding them different distances apart to see where the current feels stronger and where it weakens. You may sense a flexible shape to the air space. Sometimes it feels as though you are holding a ball between your hands.

The more you relax and direct your breathing down your arms, the stronger the sensation will become. You will notice that this process releases tension in your shoulders and arms.

You can use this directed breathing to relax tight muscles in other parts of your body as you move. Being able to send this energy to different parts of your anatomy gives you a resource for reviving tired muscles and spirits.

Lotions and Potions

The essential oils suggested for use in treatments for different body parts are selected for several key reasons. Many oils and scents known to have medicinal effects on specific health conditions also can produce allergic reactions from time to time. However, the oils selected in these chapters have been tested by herbalists to be nontoxic, non-irritating, and nonsensitizing when used in normal, nonexcessive doses. Each oil is also selected for its specific healing effect on the body area featured in that chapter. These essential oils are compatible with homeopathy and can be used both for their scent and as a lubricant. Several drops mixed into a light vegetable oil, such as almond, creates a massage oil scented to your aromatic taste.

A fifteen-minute massage increases alertness and performance. After massage, office workers complete math tests more quickly and with fewer errors.

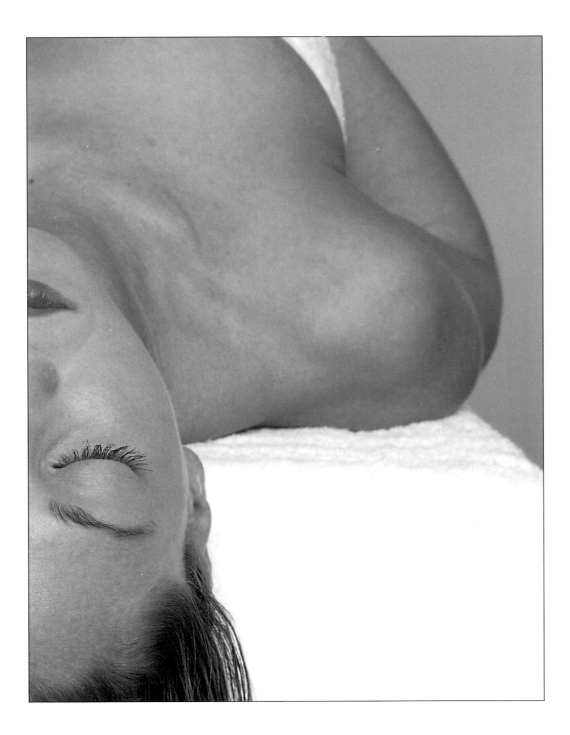

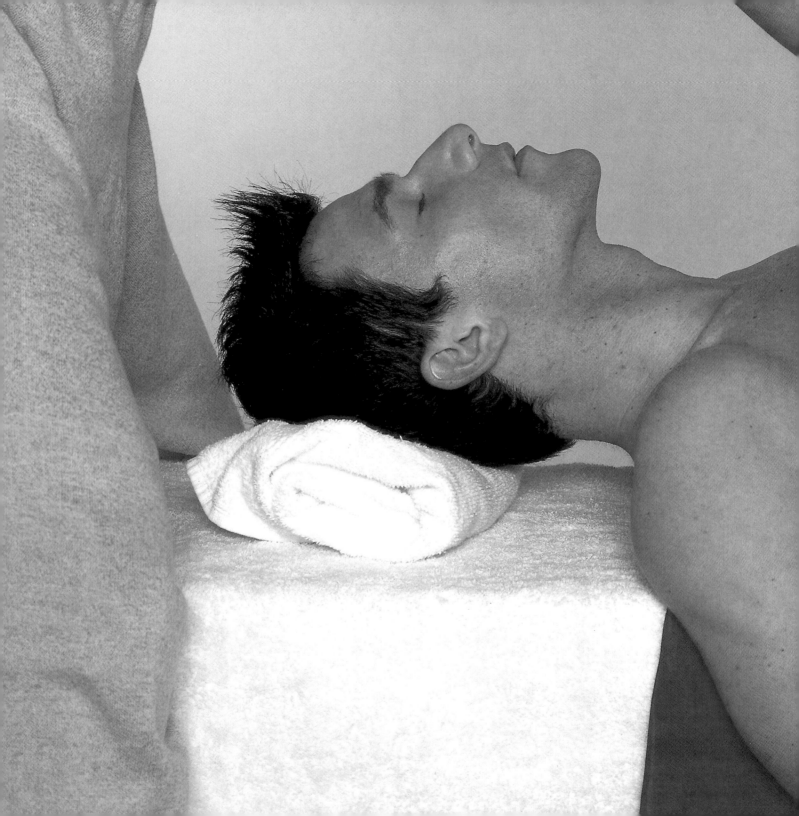

The Seven Centers
of Health

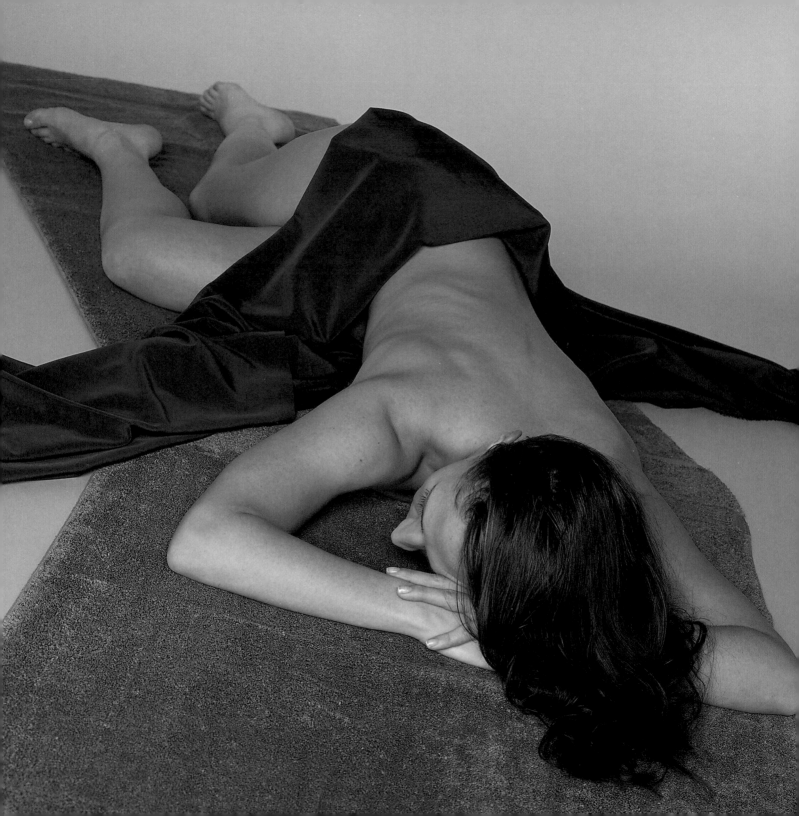

Pelvic Plexus

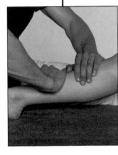

The Pelvic Plexus is centered in the lower back, the pelvis, the genitals, the legs, and the feet, and includes the kidneys and the adrenal organs.

Spirit Spa:
Meditation on Security

- Psychological associations: relationship to family, sense of stability and vitality.

- Massage for lower back, sacrum, legs, and feet.

- The healing element is earth. The symbolic color is green.

- Healing scents and oils include lavender vera, East Indian sandalwood, patchouli, Canadian balsam, jasmine, rosewood, and damask rose.

My Feet, My Roots

Psychologically, the feet represent our relationship to the earth. In more detail, this association includes our attitudes about our roots, our mothers and fathers, our sense of solidity and reality. The feet affect how secure we feel about life's basic necessities, home, family, law, and social order. These basics affect our sense of security and our ability to stand up for ourselves. Just as a strong foot represents a solid stand in the face of life's adversities, an injured foot represents a chink in our powers. Even the great warrior Achilles found out that a weak heel can be deadly.

> *To stand upright, humans balance on three points of the foot that touch the ground: the heel and the outer and inner edges of the ball of the foot.*

Care of the feet, such as washing and grooming, represents respect for a person's basic nature. A foot massage from a friend is a gift of support and acceptance.

Physiologically, feet are an extremely intense zone because nerve threads from all over the body culminate there. Thus foot massage can relax nerves and send renewed energy to all parts of your body. Structurally, feet are essential to the support of the standing body. This function associates feet with our ability to be physically as well as spiritually "upright." When you feel like running away but have to stand your ground, a foot rub can help renew your resolve and courage.

The leg also helps a person stand erect, and thus is a symbol of firmness, support, founding, erecting, and raising to new heights.

Lavender Vera Aromatherapy

Using lavender vera oil as an aromatherapy scent is a well-established folk remedy for nervous tension, shock, vertigo, and depression. The oil helps cure athlete's foot, insect bites, and muscular aches and pains such as lumbago. Because the lavender vera plant is very aromatic, planting it near your windows and doors can be healing. The plant prefers a climate with cold winters and hot summers and a full-sun location.

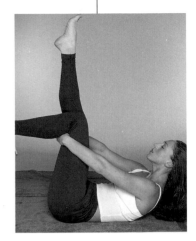

Security Meditation

You may light a candle or heat an essential oil incense with one of the healing scents for this chakra. Sit comfortably cross-legged or in full lotus on a mat on the floor. Place a small pillow or rolled towel under your tailbone to tilt you forward so that you can sit easily upright without tensing your back muscles.

Silently ask yourself one or more of these questions to increase your awareness of your sense of security and how to nourish it. Allow all of the answers to surface and then fade until no more answers come. Then move on to the next question. Close your meditation with a question that encourages strengthening your sense of security.

Do I feel part of a loving, supportive family?
Do I feel I can take care of myself well?
Do I stand up for my beliefs and desires?
Do I act as part of a supportive family for my loved ones?
How can I improve my sense of secure strength
    and family support today?

AUM Meditation

Reality in yoga is the perspective beyond our personal viewpoint when we feel unity with the divine and see everything as part of this spirit. Yoga divides our average, muddled mind-sets into three categories—waking, dreaming, and unconscious—all of which present distorted views of reality. The AUM chant (OM is the phonetic English spelling) is an exercise designed to trigger a peaceful perspective through the repetition of sacred symbolic sounds of three Sanskrit letters that stand for:

A: the self in the material world
U: the dream or psychic realm
M: the unknown conscious

Sit comfortably with your eyes closed for one to twenty minutes and repeat "AUM." Chanting these letters together as the sound OM can help unite our perceptions so that we experience a sense of our place in the larger cosmic order. We realize we are part of a huge global and universal family. Wherever we are, we have roots, we are home.

Skin is the human body's largest organ, accounting for 18 percent of our body weight and covering about nineteen square feet.

Body Spa:
Foot and Leg Massage

Sandalwood and Rose Massage Oil

- 1   cup cold-pressed almond oil
- 3   drops East Indian sandalwood essential oil
- 2   drops damask rose essential oil

Combine the oils in a plastic squeeze bottle. Sandalwood oil is soothing and moisturizing to the skin. East Indian sandalwood is superior to other forms of sandalwood for herbal treatments. The scent helps relieve sore throat, nausea, and stress depression. Damask rose oil helps erase wrinkles and improves circulation. The scent relieves uterine and genital disorders and raises the feeling of well-being.

Oatmeal and Marigold Oil Foot Paste

- 4   drops marigold essential oil
- 1/4   cup dry organic oatmeal
- 1/4   cup ground almonds
- 2   tablespoons almond oil
- 2   tablespoons honey

Before bedtime, mix ingredients together in a glass or ceramic bowl. Rub paste onto feet and then put on cotton socks. Allow the paste to soak on feet overnight. In the morning, remove socks and rinse feet in room temperature to cool water. This paste is a gentle exfoliant and moisturizer. Pure asterac marigold oil is renowned for its skin-healing properties. The paste can also be used on the hands or on any other area that needs old skin removed.

Zone Therapy*

The principle of Zone Therapy is that for every organ or muscle area in the body there is a spot that corresponds to it on one or both feet. To treat a health problem affecting the rest of the body you can massage the corresponding area on the foot. As a supplement to medical attention, Zone Therapy can provide a helpful health boost.

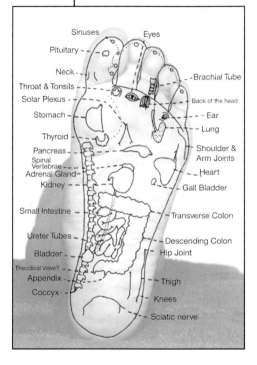

The sole of your friend's foot should be easily accessible to you. If you are working on a massage table, and your friend lies on his or her back, you sit or stand facing the sole of the foot. Massage the sole of the foot with the tips of your thumbs. Press as hard as is comfortable to your friend.

Massage the entire sole slowly and thoroughly. You may lift the foot slightly to work the sides of the heel and the ankle. If you already know of a health problem, go to the corresponding area of the foot and work there in a concentrated way for a while. Otherwise, if you find an unusual muscular constriction, lump, or reaction of pain on the part of your friend, check the Zone Therapy chart to determine what body part corresponds to the sore area. Let your friend know that there is a possible health problem related to that particular part. Massage the sore area on the foot thoroughly but without causing pain. Pain will cause more stress and tension—the opposite of your goal.

Treatments of ten to twenty minutes once a day or every two days are best for someone with a health problem. Continue this program until the condition has improved and the soreness is gone when you massage the foot.

Foot Massage

You may do foot muscle massage along with Zone Therapy or as a separate treat. Spread oil on the foot. Form a fist with your right hand. Steady the foot with your left hand. With the knuckles of your right hand, massage the sole. Press fairly hard and slide your knuckles in small circles. Cover the entire sole, including the bottom of the heel.

Foot Definition

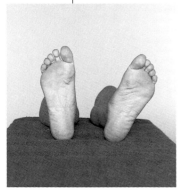

On the top of your friend's foot, find the long thin tendons running to each toe. Glide the tip of your thumb firmly down each valley that lies between the tendons. Begin at the base of the ankle and end at the small web of skin between the toes. Gently squeeze the web by pressing the tip of your forefinger against its underside as your thumb slides over its top. This flourish adds a sense of completion to the definition of the foot.

Ankle Inside Point*

The area around the ankle feels good to massage, but one spot under the ankle bone has particular relaxation punch. You can benefit from deep pressure here, so position your fingers to press hard with your thumbs.

> *Every individual has a characteristic, identifiable field of electric charge.*

Under the ankle bone is a tiny tendon. Press under the tendon and lift up toward the ankle bone. Hold this lift and exert pressure. Start lightly and increase the pressure as any soreness there dissolves. Release very gradually.

Repeat on the other foot. This is a key acupuncture point that reaches many areas of the body. Hold the pressure as long as you can and you will be rewarded in tension release.

Sole Revival*

Massaging a Japanese Shiatsu point on the foot can increase general energy and vitality. Place your thumb or forefinger just below the ball of the foot at the center of the sole. Apply firm pressure into the groove. Wait to feel how your friend's foot responds, and if it is comfortable, press more deeply. Rather than sliding, hold a steady pressure in one spot for about fifteen seconds. Release gradually.

Toe Squeezes

Steady the top of your friend's foot with your left hand. Grasp the base of the big toe with the thumb and forefinger of your right hand. Then gently pull as you slide your thumb and forefinger off the tip of the toe. Treat each toe in turn.

Next begin again with the big toe, but this time when you pull downward, twist around to the right in a corkscrew motion to give each toe a relaxing spiral stroke.

Foot Fold

Securely hold the foot with the heels of both your hands against the top and your fingertips, touching one another, pressing into the middle of the sole. Begin pressing quite hard downward on the top of the foot with the heels of your hands and upward into the sole with your fingertips. Now slowly allow the heels of your hands to slide out to either edge of the foot. Reaching the edge, keep your fingertips in place as you position the heels of your hands back in the center of the top of the foot to begin the stroke again. Repeat this stroke several times on each foot.

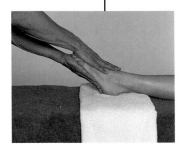

Foot Sandwich

A fine finish to the foot massage is the comforting Foot Sandwich. Place one of your palms along the sole of your friend's foot and the other along the length of the top. For several moments allow yourself to be still. Notice your breathing and relax it deeper into your abdomen. Imagine that you can breathe into your hands. What would it feel like if you could allow the energy that circulates in your body to send warmth and relaxation into the person you are massaging?

Leg Main Stroke

Position your friend's feet about a foot apart. Spread oil over the entire front and sides of the right leg. Stand near your friend's right foreleg and turn about halfway toward the opposite end of the table, facing the hips. Shift your weight onto your right foot and slide your left foot several feet toward the head of the table.

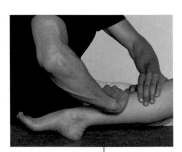

On your friend's ankle, position your right hand with fingertips facing toward you. Position your left hand snug in front of the right with fingertips facing the opposite side of the table. (Later, when working on the left leg, the right hand will go in front of the left hand.) Cup both hands, keeping your fingers together and keeping the thumb of the left hand close against the little finger of the right so that your two hands form a continuous surface with which to massage.

Begin moving your hands slowly, firmly, and steadily from one end of the leg to the other, moving slowly over the knee. When you want to apply more pressure, lean over the leg so that you use your own weight rather than an increased muscular tension. Shift your weight from your right to your left foot as you massage up the leg. Pace the speed of the two hands as they divide at the top of the leg so that they end up parallel to one another as they head downward. To do this, the inside hand must move more slowly than the outside.

When you reach the top of your friend's leg, your hands separate. The left hand continues upward to define the hip bone. Then it outlines the hipbone all the way down to the table, the fingertips applying slightly more pressure as they edge the curve of the bone.

When the fingertips touch the table, the left hand begins to glide down the side of the leg back toward the foot. At the same time, the right hand glides more slowly down the inside of the thigh. The fingertips follow the natural crease in the skin between the pelvis and the inside of the thigh, but detour around the genitals, down to the table.

The right hand also begins to head back down the leg. As you shift your weight back onto your right foot, glide your hands along the sides of the legs down to the ankle. Use lighter pressure than when massaging upward, but let your friend enjoy a firm pull as your hands slide down.

At the ankle, be sure to place your left hand higher up on the foreleg than your right. This will keep the hands from being in each other's way when they divide. (And later when you move to your friend's left leg, you'll need to position your right hand above your left on that ankle.) Repeat the Leg Main Stroke several times.

Acupuncture increases red blood cell production for up to six weeks.

Knee Circles

Start with your two thumbs crossed under the knee. Simultaneously bring both thumbs up either side of the kneecap. Then allow them to cross at the top. Finish by drawing each thumb down the side opposite from which it started. At the base of the kneecap, cross the thumbs again to be in position to begin another circle. Glide through several slow circles without stopping or lifting your thumbs.

Knee Palms*

With the palms and fingers of both hands moving at once, make several wide circles on opposite sides of the knee to relax the leg muscles there.

Acupressure Tendon Revival*

This is a key pressure point for all tendon and muscle problems and is great for athletes or people who spend a lot of time on their feet. Stimulation here can improve circulation in the body, balance liver functioning, and help heal muscle and tendon tears and strains. It also improves digestion. The spot is about four finger widths below the kneecap on both legs, on the outer side of the leg, in the valley between the two bones of the shin (tibia and fibula). You and your friend will know when you've found it because pressure there feels more intense than other spots nearby. Press with one finger or thumb and exert steady pressure for up to thirty seconds. Release gradually.

Calf and Thigh Squeezes

Be sure the leg is well oiled for this one. Cup both palms around one ankle. Your thumbs are on top of the leg. Your fingers are underneath. The general stroke is to press your fingertips firmly up into the leg from underneath and hold the pressure for a count of about two. Loosen your grip to release the deep pressure while maintaining full hand contact on the leg. Then shift your pressure onto your thumbs and quickly rotate them toward and past each other several times in a circular wringing motion on top of the leg. Now release the thumb pressure a bit. Inch your cupped hands up the leg to a new spot and repeat this squeezing and circling there. Continue up the leg to about halfway up the thigh. Press lightly behind the knee, and deeper on large muscles.

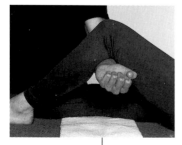

Double-Leg Main Stroke

The main stroke up both legs at once is a wonderful finale to a fine leg and foot massage. Ask your friend to lie prone. Standing at one side of the table near your friend's shins, lean over the table slightly. Start with your right hand, fingers pointing inward, across the back of your friend's right ankle. Your left hand, fingers pointing inward, is placed across the back of the left ankle. Glide up both legs at once, then over the buttocks and all the way up the back. You will need to walk a few steps to cover this area.

Now glide down the body, pulling both hands down the sides of the torso, over the hips, and down the outer sides of both legs, and even onto the feet. Try to exert equal pressure with both hands so that the receiver feels even touch all the way up and down the body. Repeat this sequence several times.

Leg Feathers*

As you come to the close of the Main Stroke, slide your hands up the leg as before, but on your way down, touch with just your fingertips as lightly as possible. Most people thoroughly enjoy this soothing stroking. If you feel your friend's top half has been left out of the relaxation process, add the Full Feathers and Claws.

Full Feathers and Claws

Using only the tips of the fingers of both hands, and touching as lightly as you can on the surface of the skin, administer a series of feather-light strokes down the neck, back, and legs, all the way to the feet. You can alternate using your fingertips with using your nails for a subtle change of texture. Finish with feather-light stroking with your fingertips.

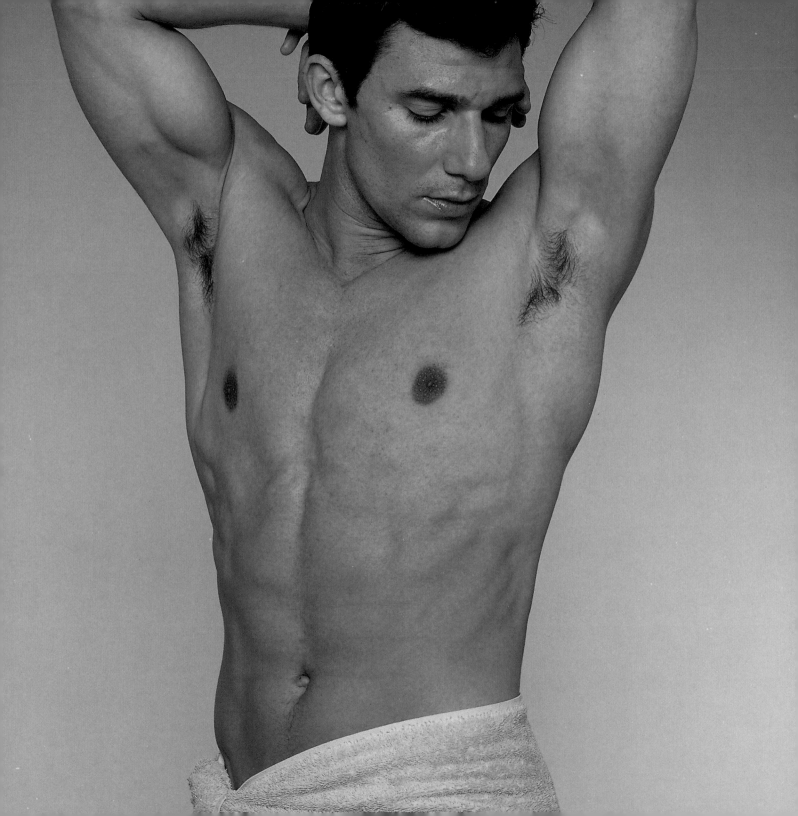

Belly Plexus

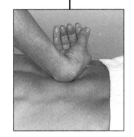

The Belly Plexus is centered in the lower back, hips, buttocks, and abdominals.

Spirit Spa:
Meditation on Control

- Psychological associations: relationship to sex, power, and responsibility.

- Massage for lower back, hips, buttocks, and abdominals.

- The healing element is water. The symbolic color is pink.

- Healing scents and oils include orange blossom, East Indian sandalwood, cardamom, lavender vera, marigold, and vetiver.

My Belly, My Center

Psychologically, the belly represents the center of our bodies, the location of balance, inner and outer, our sense of individual solidity. The pelvis is the round bowl that holds it. The belly is the place of digestion and thus a symbol of transformation of matter into more fluid substances, of bringing exterior material inside to change it into nourishment, food for the soul. Since the belly is round and the planets and atmosphere are around it, the belly with its central navel is a symbol of the concentric circles of heaven and earth. In every culture, diagrams of the universe show concentric circles with a dot at the center representing God, or the Creator, the pure principle of the universe. Meditating on your navel represents bringing your focus to the point of unity with the Divine.

There are five million touch receptors in our skin that send messages along the spinal cord to the brain.

Vetiver Aromatherapy

Vetiver is known in Sri Lanka and India as "the oil of tranquillity." The scent is effective in massage oils and bath oils to relax nervous tension and muscular aches and relieve depression and stress. It soothes sprains, stiffness, and muscle pains.

Meditation on Control

You may light a candle or incense with one of the healing scents of this chakra. Sit comfortably on a mat on the floor, with your knees bent and legs crossed in a loose lotus position. Place a small pillow or rolled towel under your tailbone to support your spine and tilt your weight slightly forward. This angle should allow you to balance and sit up straight without having to tense your back muscles. The head, neck, and torso are in a straight line, while the lower back is slightly arched.

Rest your hands, palms up, on your knees. Touch your thumb to the forefinger to form a loose circle. Close your eyes. Relax your breathing so that you can feel movement low in the muscles of your abdomen as you puff out (inhale) and sink in (exhale). If you can do so comfortably, reposition your legs into a full lotus (knees bent, ankles crossed on top of each other). Otherwise remain in a loose lotus.

Visualize that your pelvic area and abdominals are warmed by a rosy light from within. Close your eyes and silently ask and answer some of these questions on control.

Do I feel comfortably in control of my life?
What do I think prevents me from feeling in control?
What helps me feel in control?
Do I have enough money to do most of the things I want to?
Do I control my own money?
Do I allow others to manipulate me with money?
Am I happy with my sex life? Am I in control of this part of my life?
What inspires my creativity?
Do I feel guilty when I enjoy my sexuality?
How can I become more creative and honorable in my
*   intimate relationships today?*

The Hara, or Center

Centering can be accomplished through various physical and mental exercises that bring opposing elements into perspective, until they are perceived realistically as parts of a whole. This process draws the disparate influences around you into a unified order by focusing your attention on one thought or picture. From the resulting state of

---

Allow the fulfillment to come to you, gently resisting the temptation to chase your dreams into the world.
— Maharishi, *Unconditional Life*

internal harmony, you can have a calm perspective to see events and emotions more clearly.

Mandala designs are visual aids for centering. Combining a seen mandala and a spoken mantra chant in your mental meditation involves multiple senses and thus intensifies the power of the centering experience.

Centering

1 Sit in a comfortable meditation posture. Place a mandala picture an inch or so below your eye level in the center of your vision, at least four feet away from you on a table or footstool. (Jose and Miriam Arguelles encourage you to paint your own meditation image in their book *Mandala*. Their book also offers pictures of many beautiful mandalas for your meditation practice.)

2 Gaze steadily at the central area of the mandala image without allowing your eyes to blink very often. Allow your breathing to stay relaxed in your lower abdomen.

3 Maintain this gaze as long as is comfortable. Even though your eyes remain focused on the center, you will notice that visual changes occur in the areas of the picture in your peripheral vision. After a while, however, your vision will become more focused on the central spot. The center symbolizes the source of life energy. Try meditating on this concept as you gaze. Notice how your thoughts and vision change as you meditate.

Meditation Squat

This position opens hip joints to release pressure on the lower back and relaxes and sensitizes the pelvis. It relieves pinching of the sciatic nerves leading from the base of the spine across the hips and down the legs.

1 With feet shoulder-width apart, bend your knees and squat. Try to keep your heels flat on the floor and parallel rather than turned out.

2 Press your elbows or forearms outward on the insides of your knees so your hip joints are stretched a bit. As you rest, your forehead can lean forward onto your clasped hands.

3 Gradually relax so that the position, rather than muscle tension, is holding you in place.

4 You can chant "AUM" in this position or silently count your breath cycles from one to ten. After counting ten cycles of inhaling and exhaling, begin again with number one.

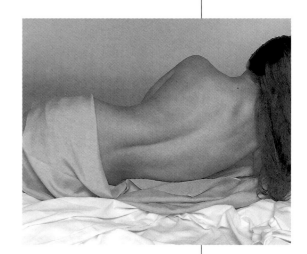

Emotions and the Back

Because of the interaction of mind and body, we need to be aware of the role of our emotions in our backs' health. Many back problems are the result of chronic daily tensions. Under prolonged stress, the body gives way eventually and the tension earns the new label: "back problem." In considering the correspondence of psychological factors to back tension, we might ask ourselves, "Why would we unnecessarily hold any part of the body tight? Why wouldn't we choose to relax and move freely?" Problems do not always spring from the fact that our bodies grow tired as we grow older, because many young people develop back problems, while many older people do not.

Folklore, psychology, and medicine all attribute certain emotional content to back problems. Many of our figures of speech reveal our assumptions about the meaning and moods of the back. For instance: "Don't turn your back on me." "You have no spine." "She shoulders too much responsibility." "I need a shoulder to cry on." "It's on your back." "He's flat on his back." "He'll back out on you." "Back off!"

In body therapy analysis, the function of a tense body part gives a clue to the cause of the problem. Sexual fears and early-childhood anxieties are often causes of lower back problems, as well as being heavy emotional burdens. Unexpressed heartfelt emotions are often held in tense chests and middle back muscles. Tight shoulders are thought to be signs of too much responsibility, unexpressed anger, or stifled ambitions.

Sadness and fear as well as the tension of unsaid words are sometimes thought to be held in tense throat muscles. A stiff neck is often thought to be a sign of opinionatedness.

Popular generalizations often prove valid. But because each body part has many functions and each person's functioning is individual, relying on the generalizations is dangerous. A person's unique patterns may be overlooked. So in psychological analysis, regard a bodily function as just one among many corresponding clues that lead to a diagnosis. Whatever its meaning, body tension must be cleared up before the psychological problem can be completely healed.

The inseparable connection of physical and emotional tension is a major reason for maintaining full body mobility. It's not only the muscles and joints that benefit from movement; the whole body and psyche are nourished by exercise. When you are properly aligned and flexible, there is more room in your body for the organs, more room for breathing. Breathing affects the circulation of blood to all the organs and tissues in the body. When your body is aligned, you not only move beautifully and more functionally, your emotional and psychological tensions are freed from their hiding places in your body and may be integrated and dealt with in the process of living.

Some doctors now refer to a type of individual as having a "backache personality." Ambition is a major giveaway of this profile, especially worldly ambition. To the backache personality, work is often an absolute priority, leading to the sacrifice of physical health in order to meet project demands. These people often think of themselves as invincible and have a "mind over matter" attitude. They also may kid themselves that they are in as good shape now as they were in their youth, when stress was never too much for their available stamina.

Besides seeing themselves as Wonder Women or Bionic Men, backache personalities may also be reluctant to appear socially distraught. Maintaining a cool veneer may seem more necessary than giving in to emotional and physical impulses. Dr. Bernard Finneson in his book *The New Approach to Low Back Pain*, writes about such sufferers:

The psychiatrist called upon to assess a patient with low back pain would look into whether the person was under stress, especially whether the person saw himself as carrying burdens beyond his capacity to bear under circumstances where the struggle involved failed to provide the gratifications which were his due or which he felt were. These particular low back pain patients are troubled by inner emotional (psychic) struggles over dependency and independence. They are divided— conscientious and yet rebellious at the same time. They say yes, but they protest with their backs.

Considering all the problems that may result from holding tension in the back, it would seem wise for us to learn to recognize our emotional symptoms early and relieve their causes before they lead to major illness. If we have conflicting responses to a situation and express only the most conservative one, perhaps we should find an appropriate place, like a psychologist's pillow or a tennis backboard, to vent the responses that we feel are too negative for polite society. In this way we can help prevent suppressed anger or frustration from overburdening our lower backs. Heavy-exertion sports or strenuous exercise is a valuable outlet for emotions too strong or violent for social exchange. We also need to acknowledge sexual conflicts and deep emotional fears openly to circumvent their becoming pent-up in our muscles.

If we are ambitious, instead of expressing it as a drive to succeed in spite of our bodies' needs, we should use it to focus on staying healthy and preventing back problems. We need to be sure not only to abandon our crutches and fantasies but also to replace them with productive, healing support images. In this way our bodies can become flexible channels enabling us to process almost any stress or surprise.

Body Spa:
Abdomen and Pelvis Massage

True Lavender Massage Oil

1   cup pure pressed almond oil
    Several drops lavender vera essential oil, to your aroma preference

Combine the oils in a plastic squeeze bottle. Almond oil is excellent for moisturizing the skin without clogging pores. True lavender oil helps soothe skin inflammations and relax muscle aches. The scent helps relieve insomnia, headache, stress, and abdominal cramps.

The largest skeletal muscle is the huge gluteus maximus, which forms the largest part of the buttock.

Abdomen Main Stroke

Stand at one end of the massage table or bed behind your friend's head. Gently position your palms down on the sternum bone in the middle of the chest with the heels of your hands resting slightly below the collarbone; fingers angled toward the feet. Glide your hands slowly forward. Apply firm pressure on the chest but lighter on the stomach.

When you reach the lower abdomen, separate your hands, moving both to the sides, and slide them down the hips to the table. When your hands touch the table, begin pulling them, heels of the hands first, along the sides of the torso up toward the shoulders. Grip firmly as you lean back, using your body weight to strengthen the pull.

Just before you reach the armpits, slide your hands onto the top of the chest just below the collarbones. Pivot each hand on its heel so the fingertips move to the center of the chest. From here you can begin another sequence of the same stroke without stopping the flow of your movement.

Here is a variation that reaches muscles on all sides of the torso. Begin in the same way. Then, when you reach the lower abdomen and slide your hands down the sides of the hips, continue to slide your hands, palms up, under the lower back. Lean way over your friend to reach as far as you comfortably can. Positioning one palm on either side of the spine, press up quite firmly with the first two fingers of each hand, into the grooves on either side of the spine between the vertebrae and the long back muscles. Pressing hard, drag your hands up these grooves near the top of the ribs, relax your fingers, and slide your hands out to the side from under the back so that you end up below the breasts on top of the ribs, with your fingers pointing toward the stomach. From here continue the abdomen massage as you did earlier in this Main Stroke.

Stomach Circles

When you massage the abdomen area, your friend's stomach will be less taut and more comfortable if the knees are bent and propped up while you are working. Lift your friend's legs under the knees and the ankles. Slide the feet closer to the hips so that the knees are bent and the legs can balance on their own.

Standing at your friend's right side, begin making slow full circles on the stomach with the palm of your left hand. It is important to move clockwise on the stomach, as the colon is wound clockwise, and the digestion moves in this direction. First pass just below the ribs, then onto the left side of the waist, then down and over a bit above the pelvic bone, then back to the right side of the torso at the waist where you began.

Keep the left hand rotating continuously. After one complete circle, add the motion of the right hand. As the left hand passes from the lower to the upper half of the stomach, the right hand begins a half circle running from hip to hip, outlining the bowl of the pelvic bone. When the right hand reaches the right hip, lift it in the air near the left hip, where it waits to repeat the same crescent stroke after the left hand has made another circle. Stroke rhythmically and evenly so that whenever the right hand is massaging, it is directly opposite the left hand. Complete a half dozen continuous circles with your left hand, adding a half circle with the right one each time. To your friend, this stroke will feel like soothing, overlapping waves.

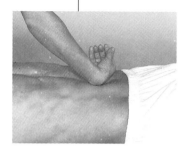

Stomach Swirls

Stand at your friend's right side. Bend your right wrist at a ninety degree angle and place the back of the hand flat against the center of the stomach, with your fingertips pointing toward you. Your forearm stands straight in the air and the elbow points away from you.

Keeping your forearm stationary, rotate your hand clockwise. After completing about a quarter of a circle, gradually turn your hand over onto its palm. Continue rotating and turning so that by the time the circle is complete, your hand is again on its back. Make several circles. This stroke should be flowing, slow, and kept to the center of the stomach.

Acupressure Stomach Balance*

These are important acupressure points for calming stomach problems, balancing the liver and spleen, soothing associated headaches, and improving circulation to these areas.

Stand to your friend's right. Position your right hand on one foot and your left hand over the abdomen. The thumb or forefinger of your right hand finds the acupressure "Liver 3" point located in the valley between the big toe and the second toe, on the flat top of the foot, just where the bones merge, before the foot curves up toward the ankle. Place your left thumb or other fingertip about three finger widths below the navel. Apply steady pressure to both points at once. Treat one foot, then keep the stomach point pressure constant while you move your right hand to treat the other foot.

Spine Pull

Slide both hands, palms up, one from one side and one from the other, under your friend's back at the waistline. Bring your fingertips to either side of the spine.

With the backs of your hands against the table, press the fingertips of both hands up as hard as you can on either side of the spine. You may even raise the middle of your friend's body up a bit. Hold for several seconds and release. Now slide your hands, still pressing but more lightly, out from under the back and onto the center of the stomach. Articulate the waistline as you go.

Moon in Abdomen

Lightly rest your right hand, palm down, on the center of the stomach just below the navel. Slide the left hand, palm up, under the back so that it is opposite your right hand. If your friend raises her back to make room for your hand, tell her to relax her weight down again. Close your eyes. Deepen your breathing. Imagine you can exhale down your arms into your palms. Visualize warmth and light flowing down your arms and circulating inside the abdomen. Tune in to any energy you feel between your palms. Imagine a full moon sphere glowing inside your friend's abdomen between your two hands. Each time you exhale, the light grows brighter. Remove your hands very slowly.

The human spine is a stack of 35 vertebrae.

Sea Salt and Orange Blossom Back Scrub

1 1/2   cups coarse sea salt
  1/4   cup orange blossom essential oil

Mix in a ceramic or glass bowl. Stand in a shower. Cover your hand with a washcloth. Dip into the bowl and, with your palm flat against your skin, spread on the paste in smooth, circular strokes. Do not press too hard. After covering the desired areas, rinse in a warm shower using a loofah or sponge. As the sea salt helps remove dead surface skin and increases circulation, the orange blossom oil helps erase scars and stretch marks. The scent balances and soothes the nervous system, as well as improves digestion.

One ton of citrus blossoms is required to produce two pounds of essential oil.

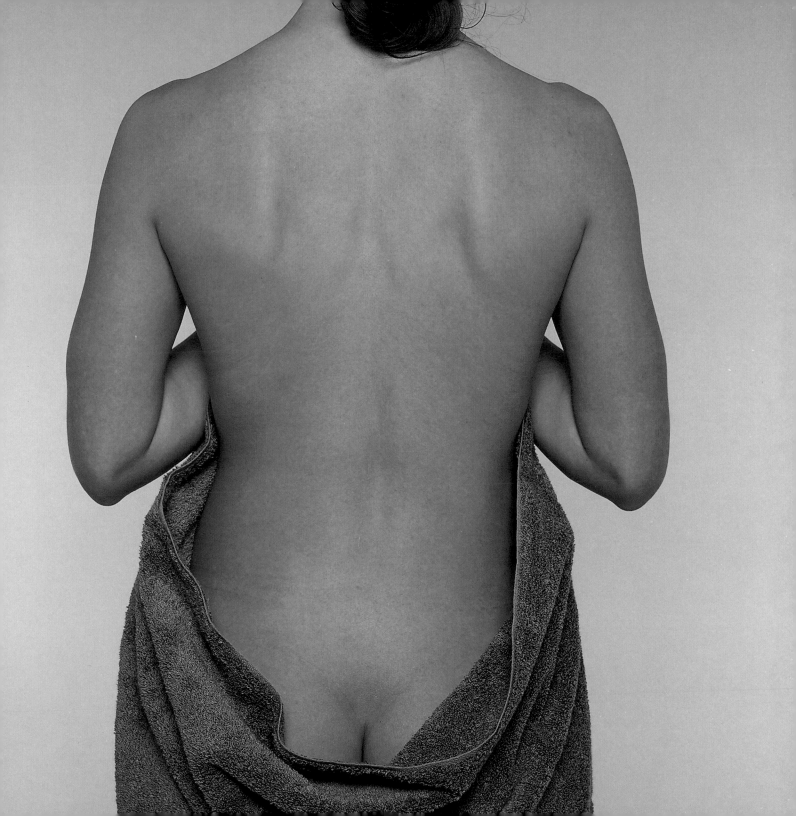

Spines through Time

Back pain causes many people trouble. A popular explanation is that human beings were never meant to walk on two legs—we were built to walk on all fours as most animals do. Certainly if we walked on four limbs, this position would release the downward pressure that is troublesome to many spines. However, we humans seem to be determined to stay upright and do all kinds of things that our backs were probably never meant to do.

Faced with the overload most of our spines carry, we need to integrate activities into our daily lives that counteract the strains of modern living and prevent us from suffering chronic aches or from resorting to complicated and painful solutions like surgery and drugs. Except in rare and urgent cases, surgery is a last resort for back and neck injuries. With the success rate of rest, therapy, and exercise treatments in most cases equaling that of surgery, which one would you choose?

In my years of experience studying and working in a variety of body therapies, I have arrived at an effective approach to healing most back pain. The massages in this book are focused on the idea that healing takes place most effectively through relaxation and pleasure. My studies in physical therapies include work in Reichian, Breyer, Proskauer, Feldenkrais, Alexander, massage, acupressure, and polarity techniques; and I spent four years on the Esalen Institute staff conducting programs in alternative treatments for medical doctors and other health professionals. During my years in private practice as a body therapist, I worked with clients who had many types of back problems. Except for those resulting from accidents, the disorders were mostly caused by a simple combination of physical and psychological tension from bad posture and emotional stress. These are areas we can treat ourselves by changing our habits, educating ourselves about our backs, and becoming more sensitive to our responses to our environment.

No matter how diverse the cases and treatments for back problems, most back specialists agree that there are three core origins of back disorders: stress, inappropriate diet, and lack of exercise. Stress often heads the list of concerns because the benefits of eating well and exercising correctly can be undermined by stress. One way to decompress is to alternate work and periods of pressure with phases of relaxation and renewal. Setting aside moments for self-care during your day is crucial to back health. Eating well consistently provides the chemical balance our bodies need to build strength and function properly at any age. Too rough and too much exercise can produce as many back problems as too little exercise. Learning to move well throughout a day's normal activities can reduce your need for separate exercise periods. Self-treatment is the focus of this book, and self-care is the most inexpensive as well as the most enduring solution to back problems.

Because establishing habits for back care, or for any body problem, is often the toughest aspect of body maintenance, the most successful treatments for backs are various forms of pleasure-oriented physical therapies, and massage is one of the most effective. Massage first focuses on relaxing injured or tense muscles so they can settle back into their proper areas, and then concentrates on rebuilding tone and strength by encouraging circulation to the area through gentle movement.

Anxiety and tension are integral parts of our modern lives. Moments of relaxation and sensitivity are the best antidotes. Nothing helps a traumatized muscle or nerve relax into place more than pleasure. Medical science has developed theories resulting from neurological research that explain aspects of this phenomenon of pleasure healing. And most of us are more likely to continue back care over time if it feels good and is fun.

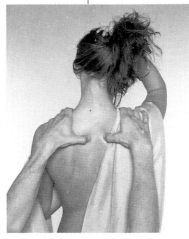

Dorology is a recently developed medical specialty devoted to the treatment of chronic pain. Pain is the body's most urgent warning signal of an imbalance. Acute pain is an alarm that we must change our condition immediately. Chronic pain is a message that we need to alter some habits in our way of life. Solving a pain puzzle can be like unraveling a many-layered mystery. Causes are not always obvious. Many routes can be explored before the original source of the pain is discovered. When the causes are obvious, sometimes the block is simply reluctance to change our behavior.

Muscles tighten, forming knots and spasms in an effort to alleviate pain. Tight muscles put pressure on blood vessels and nerves and decrease blood flow to the area. Ischemic pain, which is local anemia caused by tissue constriction, sets up a cycle of increasing tension and pain responses. The goal of most pain treatments is to short-circuit this escalating cycle.

While a variety of pain control techniques are used by dorologists, a relatively new theory called "gate control" is one of the more interesting. This theory assumes that the spinal cord acts as a "pain gate" that can be closed to prevent pain signals from reaching the brain. Pain impulses travel along both A-delta and C nerve fibers to reach the two bundles of nerve fibers on either side of the spine. If these impulses succeed in reaching the brain stem and the thalamus, they are perceived as pain. Special techniques such as acupuncture, acupressure massage, and hypnosis or meditation can change the impulses along the spinal cord to close the "gate" to the brain stem and can significantly relieve pain in many cases.

The body produces natural opiates that relieve pain. Production of these enkephalins can be triggered electrically as well as through acupuncture, acupressure, and some forms of massage. Through focused meditation and self-massage of acupressure points, we can often relieve pain and increase production of enkephalins ourselves.

The most effective solutions to our physical aches and pains come as we add preventive relaxation moments to our lives, as we think of healing less as a profession and more as a way of life. The mental state of healing is the opposite of the stages of stress and force. Replacing surgery, medication, and manipulation, the long-lasting aspects of healing are relaxation, sensitivity, and equilibrium. These are the new experts.

Hip Circles

Standing at your friend's left side, begin by forming a special hand position. Group the middle three fingers of your right hand (or left if you are left-handed) tightly together. They form a triangle with the middle finger on top. Place these three fingertips just below your friend's waistline to the right of the spine. Pressing firmly, begin moving your fingertips in circles about a half-inch wide as you slowly guide your massaging hand across the body toward the opposite side.

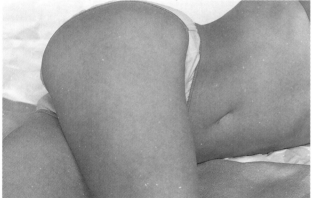

Continue making these circles, moving straight across and then down the side of the lower back, until your fingers reach the table. With almost no pressure, glide the fingertips back up the same area.

> *Six pairs of nerves from the sacrum and coccyx control your pelvic organs and buttock muscles.*

Massage down the waist, hip, and buttock in this manner. Each strip begins about an inch farther down the back or hip. Start each one just beside the spine; then slide back up the same strip once your fingers have reached the table. Work all the way down the right buttock. Then cross to the other side of the table to massage the left lower back and buttock muscles.

Kneading the Buttocks

Knead the muscles of either buttock by lifting the flesh and squeezing it between the thumb and your other fingers. Massage rhythmically, alternating hands. Massage the other buttock in the same alternating strokes.

Buttocks Shake

If you and the person you are massaging can overcome the feeling that you are doing something silly, you'll discover a new, relaxing treat for the lower back and hips. Spread the fingers of your right hand as wide apart as possible. Position your hand firmly centered against the lower curves of both buttocks at once. Now shake your hand lightly but very quickly from side to side, vibrating the buttocks beneath your hand.

Lower Back Thumb Rolls

This stroke feels terrific on the upper back, on the lower back, and just about anywhere there's a muscle in need of soothing, rhythmic pressure. The Thumb Roll stroke is especially relaxing to the overstressed lower back muscles. Standing behind your friend's head, lean over the back and locate the top of the arrowhead-shaped bone, the sacrum, at the base of the spine. (The "arrow" points toward the feet.) Alternating thumbs, slide your thumbs away from you in short, rapid strokes. Concentrate on the small but crucial strips of muscle on top of the sacrum. Work down to the base of the spine. Then continue your Thumb Rolls across one hip and then down the other. The large hip muscles will enjoy deeper work.

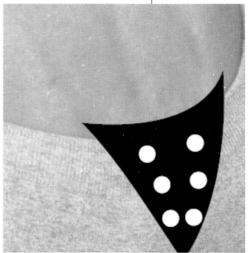

Pelvis Pressure Points*

These pressure points are used for releasing lower back and pelvis tension in Shiatsu treatment, a form of Japanese pressure-point massage based on the same energy system as acupuncture. Although the complete system requires training, you can use a simple version of pressure-point massage for relaxing effects.

Place your palms on top of your friend's lower back. Locate the top edge of the sacrum. Lean your weight into your arms as you press your thumbs on either side of one of your friend's sacral vertebrae. As you feel the muscles under your thumbs relax and soften a bit, very gradually angle more of your weight into your hands.

Release the pressure just as gradually as you applied it, so that your hands come out of your friend's muscles very slowly. Then move your thumbs down to the next sacral vertebrae. Apply the pressure of your body weight again. Work your way from the top of the sacrum to the tip. Then apply the same type of gradual pressure to the outsides of the sacrum, from your friend's waist down to the tailbone. The pressure should be deep but not painful. If it is painful you are pressing either too quickly or too hard for her muscles to relax with the pressure. You might not be in quite the right spot, so shift your position and try another spot.

To press on your own sacrum points, lie on one side with your knees bent and folded up toward your chest. Reach behind and use the thumb of your upper hand to press on your sacrum points.

Full Body Strokes

A soothing way to end a massage is with a few strokes running up and down the full length of the body. Such strokes will leave your friend with an awareness of his or her body as a connected whole.

Using a light touch with all your fingertips, stroke down the length of the back, over the buttocks, and all the way down one leg. Start at the shoulders again and stroke down the back, the buttocks, and all the way down the other leg.

A nerve impulse takes .000,001 percent of a second to cross a synapse.

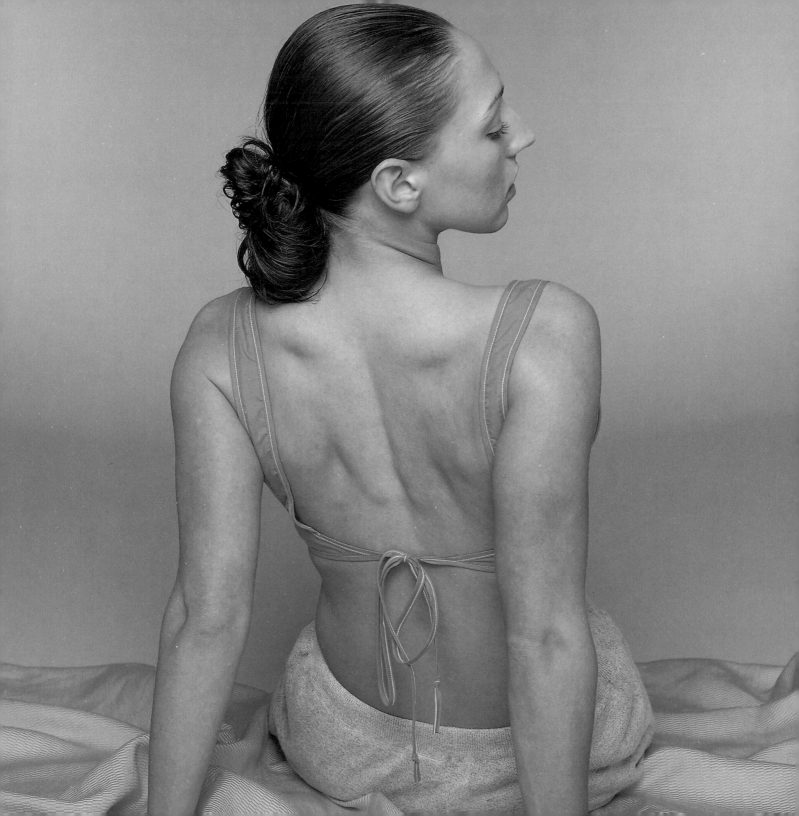

Solar Plexus

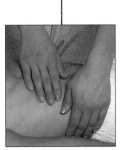

The Solar Plexus is centered in the chest and diaphragm region.

Spirit Spa:
Meditation on Trust

- Psychological associations: self-confidence, respect for self and others, relationships to fear and external power.

- Massage for torso and chest.

- The healing element is fire. The symbolic color is orange.

- Healing scents and oils include cypress, vetiver, mimosa, damask rose, and jasmine.

My Diaphragm, My Ego

Psychologically, the diaphragm area at the base and center of the ribs is the seat of the ego and houses our sense of outer-directed power. It is the spot in the center of our chest to which most of us point when we want to indicate "I." Comfort or problems in this area are symbolically related to external power, to how we present ourselves to the public, to our sense of self-confidence and respect for ourselves as well as for others. Since fear undermines self-confident presentation, the Meditation on Trust focuses on calming anxieties and nurturing a sense of inner strength and confidence. The Baby Massage is included in this chapter because babies represent our trust in the future, our confidence in ourselves, and our ability to be trusted by someone else.

> *The twelve spinal vertebrae just below the neck extend around the torso of the body to form the rib cage that protects the heart and lungs.*

Italian Cypress and Asian Jasmine Aromatherapy

Italian cypress helps strengthen the functioning of the liver and the respiratory system, increases circulation, and calms nervous tension. Jasmine is soothing to the liver and the skin, and is traditionally thought to promote feelings of optimism and confidence.

Rose Milk Bath

1 cup dried milk powder
5 drops damask rose essential oil
   Petals of one rose blossom
   Peel of one orange, cut into thin strips

When the water for a comfortably hot bath is about half drawn, slowly pour the dried milk flakes under the running water. Add the rose oil and orange peel. When the bath is full, sprinkle the rose petals on top of the water. Soak and dream of Cleopatra. The milk's protein is good for your skin. Citrus improves circulation. Scent of damask rose bolsters confidence and raises spirits.

Meditation on Trust

You may heat an essential oil incense or light a candle with the scent of one of the healing herbs for this body area.

Sit in a comfortable lotus position on a mat on the floor. Place a candle in front of you on a low table or stand so that the top of the candle is level with your eyes as you sit. Light the candle. Circle your thumb to your forefingers, and rest each hand, palm up, on the knee. Gaze steadily at the flame without blinking for about one minute. Then close your eyes, relax the muscles, and visualize an orange flame glowing between your eyebrows.

Alternate periods of flame-gazing with open eyes and flame-visualizing with closed eyes for periods of up to three minutes. Develop your gaze gradually. Do not strain your eyes. This sequence builds concentration and strengthens the nerve centers.

Each time you meditate, you may focus on one aspect of your emotional issues related to the powers of this body area. Silently ask yourself the question. Allow an answer to surface. Note it mentally. Then let the answer dissolve and allow another answer to the question surface. Continue this process until no more answers appear. Try to end your meditation with a question that encourages you to live more fully today.

What does trust mean to me?

Whom do I trust? Why?

Whom do I mistrust? Why?

Do I trust myself? Why?

Can others trust me? Why?

What fears interfere with my trusting others?

*How can I nurture my self-respect and self-confidence so that my ability
    to trust and be trusted will grow?*

How do I define honor?

How can I live more honorably today?

Visualize a warm orange light inside your chest at the center base of your ribs. Allow the light to grow stronger.

Prana

Prana is the Indian name of the energy that moves through the spinal cord and stimulates the various nerve plexus centers. When it rises up to the head, it produces intense states of mental clarity and physical balance. The ultimate aim of all breathing exercises is to raise the prana energy, called *kundalini,* to the top of the head in order to create mental and spiritual balance.

> *Premature babies who received three massages a day for ten days will gain weight 47 percent faster than nonmassaged babies. They also get out of the hospital six days sooner, sleep more deeply, and are more alert, calm, and responsive.*

Vishnu Mudra

This breathing pattern helps clear your air passages, improve your control and discrimination, and bring more life energy and oxygen though your body. Specific fingers are used because of their differing magnetic charges. Repeat the sequences several times.

1 Sit comfortably with the tip of your spine on a small pillow. Keep your legs crossed in front of you. Raise your right hand so the palm is toward your face. Fold down your index finger and the next finger.

2 Press your thumb to close your right nostril, and inhale with your left nostril to a count of four. Exhale to a count of eight. The exhalation should take twice as long as the inhalation.

3 Now release your thumb and press your left nostril closed with your ring and little fingers as you inhale through your right nostril to a count of four. Then exhale to a count of eight.

Alternate Nostril Breath

This breathing pattern helps calm the nerves and improve circulation. It is a general balancer and purifier of the physical and emotional systems. Practice prepares you for more advanced techniques.

1 Close your right nostril with your thumb. Inhale through your left nostril to a count of four.

2 Now pinch your ring and little fingers against your left nostril so both sides are closed. Hold your breath to a count of sixteen.

3 Release your thumb and exhale to a count of eight through your right nostril.

4 Next inhale through your right nostril to a count of four.

5 Pinch both nostrils closed to a count of sixteen.

6 Release your last two fingers so that you can exhale through your left nostril to a count of eight. Repeat the whole cycle several times.

Body Spa:
Torso Massage

Jasmine and Vetiver Massage Oil

1 cup pure almond oil
2 drops Asian jasmine essential oil
2 drops vetiver essential oil

Combine the oils in a plastic squeeze bottle. These scents calm anxiety and encourage confidence. The oils moisturize and soothe the skin.

Torso Main Stroke

Stand at one end of the massage table or bed behind your friend's head. Gently place your hands palms down on the sternum bone in the middle of the chest. The heels of your hands rest slightly below the collarbone; thumbs touching, your fingers point toward the feet. Now glide your hands slowly together between the breasts and down the rib cage, then over the abdomen. Apply firm pressure to the chest but use a much lighter touch on the stomach.

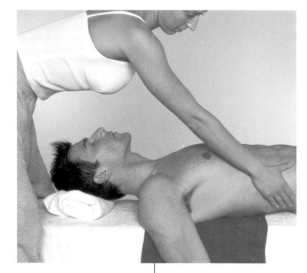

When you reach the lower abdomen, separate your hands, moving both to the sides, and slide both hands down the hips to the table. When your hands touch the table, begin pulling them, heels of the hands first, along the sides of the torso up toward the shoulders. Grip firmly as you lean back, using your body weight to strengthen the pull.

Just before you reach the armpits, slide your hands onto the top of the chest just below the collarbones. Pivot each hand on its heel so the fingertips move to the center of the chest. From here you can begin another sequence of the same stroke without stopping the flow of your movement.

To help make this stroke feel wonderful, move at a steady, confident pace. Mold your hands so that they snugly fit all contours, as if you were molding the body out of clay.

Here is a variation that includes the midback in this stroke. When you pull your hands back onto the upper chest, slide them down the sides of the shoulders, and then under the ribs below the shoulder blades. Your hands will be between the table and the back, beside but not on the spine. Now press up with your fingers and slide them along the muscles on either side of the spine, over the shoulders, and then back onto the upper chest. You are now in position to begin the Torso Main Stroke again.

Collarbone Outline*

Standing behind your friend's head, rest your palms lightly on the shoulders. Place the thumb on the upper side of the collarbone near the base of the neck and the forefinger on the lower, using both your hands. Be careful not to apply any pressure to the inch-wide indentation in the throat between the inner tips of the collarbone. Pinch slightly and slide both sets of fingers away from each other along the collarbone. When you reach the shoulder bones, lift your fingers and immediately replace them where you started. Repeat this stroke several times.

Side Pulls

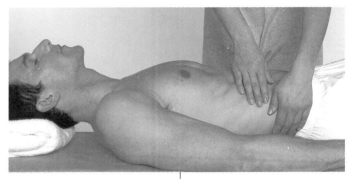

Standing to one side of the table, reach across to the opposite side of your friend's torso. Pull each hand, fingers pointing down, straight up from the table. Alternating hands, begin sliding one hand up just before the other is about to finish its pull so that there is no break between strokes. Begin pulling on the side of the hip just above the thigh and work your way up to the armpit, then back again. Move slowly, steadily, and just the width of one of your hands with each stroke.

When you are ready to massage the other side, keeping hand contact, walk to the other side of the table and repeat the Side Pulls on your friend's other side.

Torso Kneading

Reaching across to the side opposite you, gently squeeze the flesh at the waistline between your thumb and fingers. Then allow it to slip from your fingers. Slide your hands a little with each stroke, left hand toward the right and right hand toward the left. Alternate hands, beginning a new stroke with one hand just before finishing with the other. Develop a slow, comfortable rhythm in which the hands are always in motion.

Waist Cinch

Slide the fingers of both hands under your friend's back at either side of the waist. Press them all the way under until the hands are pointing toward each other just to either side of the spine. Draw your hands back out and onto the stomach as you follow the waistline and press with the fingertips. Repeat several times, lifting slightly as you pull.

Complete Sweep

This stroke offers a simple way to connect all the different strokes you've done to give your friend a delicate sense of physical unity. Rest your palms on your friend's shoulders. Lightly move your fingertips down the arms and hands and then over the hips. Now glide them down the legs to the feet. At this point, angle your hands away from each other and lift them off the body. Return your palms to the shoulders and repeat the sweep.

Baby Massage Technique

In Chinese acupuncture, health is ensured by the balance of yin and yang elements in the body. Yin is the system of the receptive aspects of the body, symbolized by the moon. Yang is the system of active elements in the body, symbolized by the sun.

The back of the body, the outsides of the legs, and the backs of the arms are considered yang. To follow the principles of acupuncture, you move your strokes down yang pathways, or meridians, and up yin meridians. This means you should move strokes along the backs of arms from shoulders to the wrists. Move strokes on the baby's back from shoulders to hips.

A Back Rub for Baby

Infants love to be massaged as much as anyone else. However, they may show their enthusiasm by moving around a lot, so you'll have to become adept at giving back rubs to a moving object. Soothing touch helps stimulate nerve and muscle development and improves coordination in infants.

Infants are in a heightened state of sensory awareness compared with adults. And sensitive massage following the shape of the body helps an infant increase the sense of self and define the boundaries between self and the rest of the world. Babies who lack touching can become depressed or ill and develop more slowly.

Back rubs are reassuring to an upset child. They can calm a child after an accident, help put the child to sleep, or simply reaffirm the bond between parent and child. A back rub for a baby should be relaxed, gentle, and in the spirit of yet another form of play shared with each other.

The infant massage techniques described here are aimed at encouraging the baby's sense of physical strength and joy, stimulating sensory and motor development, and increasing the positive bonding between parent and child.

Snug as a Bug

The baby may be massaged in any position that is comfortable for both of you. You might hold the baby against your chest while sitting and stroke the back. You can rest the baby on his or her stomach across your lap; or have the baby lie with feet toward you, on his or her stomach on your outstretched legs. Be sure to always support the baby with one hand as you massage with the other.

> *With 430,000 premature births in America each year, hospitals could save up to four billion dollars annually with baby massage treatment.*

Oils and Powders

French clay baby powder makes a pleasant massage lubricant. Pure vegetable oil, warmed in your palm before using, can also feel wonderful. Stroking lightly without oil or powder can be soothing too, if you move very gently. Or you can stroke with a pure cotton pad. Some babies also enjoy the tickle of a very soft baby brush.

Spearmint Baby Massage Oil

1/2   cup pure almond oil
2   drops spearmint essential oil

Combine oils in a plastic squeeze bottle. Almond oil is light, easily absorbed, and soothing to sensitive skin. Spearmint aroma and oil have healing properties similar to those of peppermint, but in a much milder form and are therefore appropriate for children's remedies. Distilled spearmint water relieves colic and indigestion. The scent is relaxing and soothes headache and nervous tension.

Baby Strokes

Health in the Chinese acupuncture system is maintained by the balance of the receptive, or yin, elements of the body, and the active, or yang, elements in the body. To follow the principles of acupuncture in massage, you move your strokes up yin pathways and down yang pathways.

To begin, stroke with your fingertips down the baby's backbone, moving from neck to buttocks. The rest of the strokes can be done in any sequence.

Stroke from the top of the head down the back of the neck; then proceed down the right side of the back. Continue your strokes down the outer back side of the right leg to the foot.

Starting at the back of the right shoulder, glide down the arm to the right hand. Stroke from the top of the head down the back of the neck, and then down the complete body length over the left side of the baby's back; smooth over the left outer side of the left leg and foot.

Glide from the back of the left shoulder down the arm to the left hand. Rest your palm in the center of the back between the baby's shoulder blades. Smooth a pattern of light, rhythmic circles with your fingertips or your palm on the baby's back. Occasionally stroke down the entire length of the spine to the baby's tailbone.

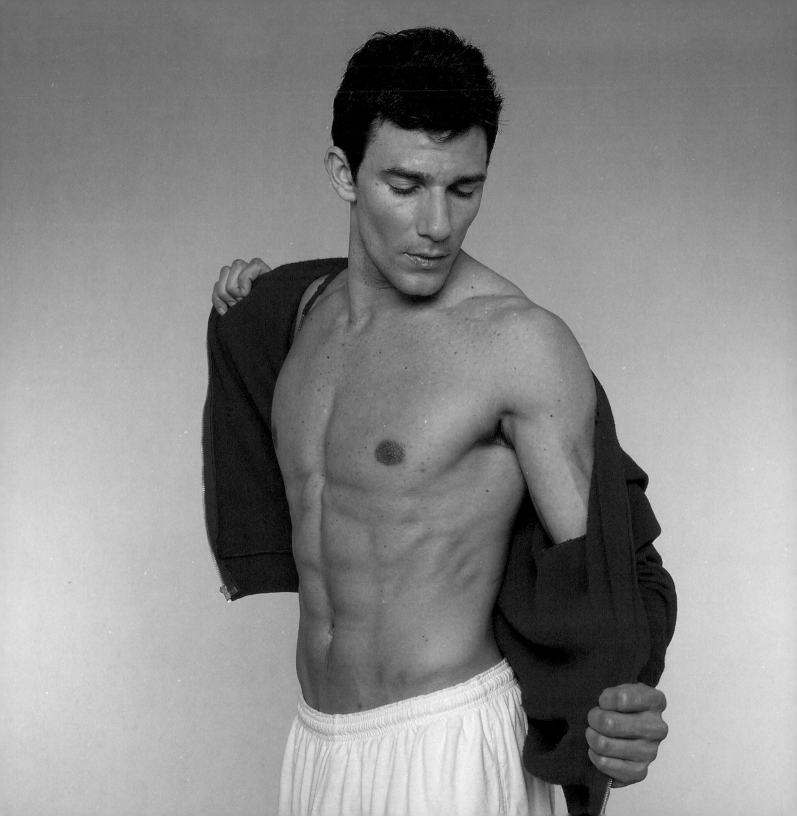

Cardiac Plexus

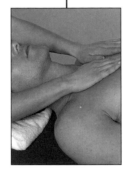

The Cardiac Plexus is centered in the chest and midback and includes the heart, the circulatory system, the lungs, the thymus gland, and the thoracic vertebra.

Spirit Spa:
Meditation on Love and Compassion

- Psychological associations: hope, forgiveness, hate, and love.

- Massage for the chest and midback.

- The healing element is air. The symbolic color is red.

- Healing scents and oils include white birch, violet, damask rose, jasmine, longleaf pine, and lime.

My Heart, My Compassion

The heart is the physical center of the blood circulation for the body and the psychological center of emotional attachment. The heart was the only organ not removed from a mummy by Egyptian embalmers, because it was regarded as indispensable in the afterlife. A heart with flames symbolizes love as the center of spiritual illumination. Because blood represents life, spilled blood represents the sacrifice of life for a noble cause. The heart is thought to be the center of passion, which, when infused with enlightened understanding, becomes compassion, or love for others.

Violet and Damask Rose Aromatherapy

The scent of violets is traditionally believed to strengthen and comfort the heart. It relieves nervousness and insomnia and improves circulation. The oil has mild painkilling properties, which are attributed to the presence of salicylic acid, the active ingredient in aspirin. Damask rose is traditionally thought to be the scent of happiness. It improves the circulation and relieves stress.

Love and Compassion Meditation

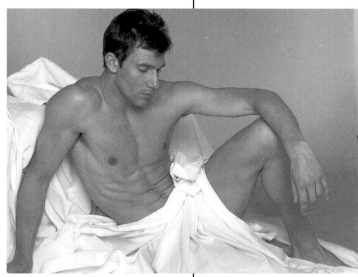

You may light a candle or heat an essential oil incense with one of the healing scents for this chakra. Sit comfortably. Relax your breathing low in your abdomen. Silently ask yourself these questions. Allow the answers to surface and pass. Notice which answers give you clues to how you block your love and compassion. Ask yourself how you can nourish them.

How do I define my love for someone?
How do I decide if someone loves me?
What responsibilities come with love?
What frightens me about love and compassion?
Am I able to forgive someone who harms me?
Am I able to set appropriate limits for demands from someone I love?
Can I experience feelings of love for wider communities
     beyond my family and friends?
What are my responsibilities to these communities?

Mantra of Compassion

Aum Mani Padme Hum Hrih
(ohm mahnee pahdmay hoom hreeh)

This mantra purifies negative emotion to transform it into our true, wise nature. It heals anxiety, negativity, confusion, and ill health, and increases our sense of compassion. Sit comfortably. Close your eyes. Repeat this sequence of sounds in a low voice as long as you comfortably can.

Aum: enlightened body
Mani Padme: enlightened speech
Hum: enlightened mind
Hrih: active compassion, propels
healing out to others

> *"The sun and moon are not mirrored in cloudy waters, thus the Almighty cannot be mirrored in a heart that is obsessed with the idea of me and mine."*
> —*Sri Ramakrishna*

Partner Yoga

Partner yoga provides a transition from your solitary practice to the application of your meditative insights to the world at large. Patterns unfolding in the interactions of each exercise offer a microcosm of your patterns of thought and behavior in wider arenas. Yoga is a doorway to more self-awareness, and partner yoga can double your insight.

|Back-to-Back Meditation|

1 Sit cross-legged, back to back with your partner. Let as much of your spines touch as possible. Find a position to rest together in which both of you are comfortable and neither feels too leaned on. Ideally, you will feel that the other person's back gives you support to sit up effortlessly.

2 Rest your hands palms up in your lap. Or you can extend both arms behind you to rest your palms on your partner's thighs. Close your eyes. Notice any movement in the muscles of your body as a result of your breathing.

3 Can you feel any movement in your partner's back as a result of his or her breathing, especially in the lower back? Can you keep aware of your own sensations while you feel another's? Notice if your breathing rhythms stay different or synchronize.

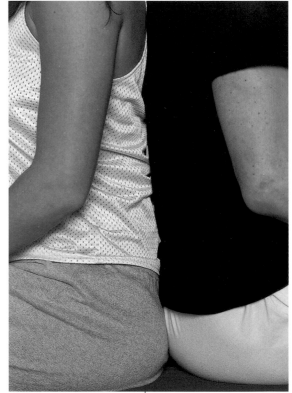

Double Palm Breathing

1 Sit cross-legged opposite your partner with your knees touching. Place your arms at your sides and your palms on your partner's palms in the following pattern. You and your partner's right palms should be facing down and the left palms facing up. The four palms fit together in mirror images. Begin by closing your eyes, relaxing your breathing, and noticing how you are feeling.

2 Now open your eyes and look into your partner's eyes. Can you continue to stay in touch with your inner feelings even when sensing someone else's? Do not try to talk or visually communicate by facial changes. Keep your expression neutral. Allow your eyes to receive and give information without censoring it. Notice if you begin to feel any sensation of an energy circuit trailing from your palms, arms, and knees to the rest of your body. Can you relax and allow this energy to flow?

3 Breathe gently through your nose. Imagine what it would feel like if you could exhale down through your body and into your arms and legs. Allow your breathing to ease tight muscles and to relax you from the inside.

4 Try imagining as you exhale that you send your breath not only down your arms but also into your palms and even into your partner's palms. What would it feel like if you could send energy to your partner as you exhale and receive energy from your partner as you inhale? Can you both give power to and accept power from your partner?

5 Now alter your position so that the soles of your feet are touching and your legs are stretched straight out between you. Keep your spine straight and your eyes in contact. Stretch your arms out about shoulder height in front of you with palms down. Your partner should also stretch out both arms, but with the palms up and hands slightly below your hands. Your four hands do not touch. Do you feel any sensation of energy exchange even though your hands are not touching now?

6 Maintaining eye contact, increase the depth and speed of your exhalation so that your abdomen contracts sharply as you exhale and the air is expelled in short, powerful bursts. This clears more stale air from the lungs and allows fresh air to come in more easily as you inhale. The faster pace speeds up your circulation. Both of you continue this fast breath to relax any aches you might feel in your muscles. Gradually slow down your breathing, relax your arms, and lie down on the floor. Allow your feet to stay touching. Rest a while.

Body Spa:
Chest and Midback Massage

Lime and Vetiver Massage Oil

1 cup pure almond oil
Several drops lime essential oil, as well as several drops vetiver essential oil, to your scent preference

Combine the oils in a plastic squeeze bottle. Lime improves circulation and relieves rheumatism. Vetiver calms and relaxes.

White Birch and Lime Bath Oil

4 drops white birch essential oil
3 drops lime essential oil
3 tablespoons olive oil

Add oils to a very warm half-full bath under the running water. Olive oil is rich in vitamins and minerals and helps balance the level of acidity in the skin. White birch relieves arthritis and muscle pain, and helps the body eliminate toxins. Lime oil improves circulation.

Chest Main Stroke

Stand at one end of the massage table or bed behind your friend's head. Gently place your hands palms down in the middle of the chest. The heels of your hands rest slightly below the collarbone; thumbs touching, your fingers point away from you. Now move your hands slowly forward. Apply firm pressure on the chest but much lighter on the stomach.

When you reach the lower abdomen, separate your hands, moving both to the sides, and slide both hands down the hips to the table. When your hands touch the table, begin pulling them, heels of the hands first, along the sides of the torso up toward the shoulders. Grip firmly as you lean back, using your body weight to strengthen the pull.

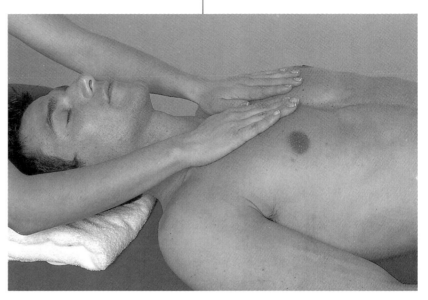

Right before you reach the armpits, slide your hands onto the top of the chest just below the collarbones. Pivot each hand on its heel so the fingertips move to the center of the chest. From here you can begin another sequence of the same stroke without stopping the flow of your movement.

To help make this stroke feel wonderful, move at a steady, confident pace. Mold your hands so that they snugly fit all contours, as if you were sculpting the body out of clay.

Here is a variation that includes the upper back in this stroke. After you pull your hands back onto the upper chest, slide them down the sides of the shoulders and then under the shoulders and onto the top part of the back. Your fingers will now be sliding between the table and the back until they are beside but not on the spine. Now slide your hands over the trapezius muscles that curve from the neck to the shoulders and upper back, and then back onto the upper chest. You are now in position to begin the Chest Main Stroke again.

Collarbone Outline*

Standing behind your friend's head, rest your palms lightly on the shoulders. Place the thumb on the upper side of the collarbone near the base of the neck, and the forefinger on the lower, using both your hands. Be careful not to apply any pressure to the inch-wide indentation in the throat between the inner tips of the collarbone. Pinch slightly and slide both sets of fingers away from each other along the collarbone. When you reach the shoulder bones, lift your fingers and immediately replace them where you started. Repeat this stroke several times.

Infinity Breasts

Named for the figure-eight-like symbol of infinity that is traced by your hands during this stroke, this is very relaxing for the often tense muscles of the upper chest. The stroke usually feels good to both women's and men's chest muscles. Standing to your friend's right, rest your right palm very lightly on the abdomen. Your left palm draws a figure eight around the breasts to massage the upper and lower support muscles.

Begin on the sternum bone between the breasts, your fingers pointing away from you. As you lean some of your weight onto your left palm, slide it around the lower edge of the left breast. Glide your hand around your friend's side, and up onto the pectoral muscles above the breast. Now move your hand, heel first, down under your friend's right breast, up her right side, and then back onto the upper chest by way of the right pectoral muscle. End up touching the place on the sternum where you began. Circle continuously around the breasts in this figure-eight pattern several times. Your right hand remains still and light on the abdomen to relax the stomach area and to balance the energy in the torso.

Ribs Opener

Standing to your friend's right, hold the wrist of his or her right arm with your left. Lift and lean the right arm to your left so that it can rest in place extended. The upper arm lies on the table beside the head and the forearm raised as if your friend is raising his hand in class. Now position both your palms lightly against your friend's armpit area, with the fingers of both hands pointing toward each other.

With a light pressure, spread your hands outward to the sides, leading with the heels of the hands. The right hand moves down the side of the torso and the left up along the upper arm. When your hands have passed the armpit itself, turn both so that they are perpendicular to the table as you keep them moving apart at an even pace.

Gently grasp the arm with your left hand, fingers on top and thumb below. Curve your right hand so that the whole palm presses against the side of the torso. In this position continue moving them apart as you increase the pressure slightly. When your right hand reaches your friend's hip and your left reaches the wrist, stop.

Keeping your hands in place, tighten your hold so that you can stretch the arm and the hip away from each other. Hold this stretch for a count of about five. Then release. Break touch contact with your friend's torso just long enough to bring your hands back to the armpit, so that you are in position to begin the stroke again. Repeat the stroke several times. Then gently place the arm back at your friend's side.

Side Pulls

Standing to one side of the table, place both hands on the opposite side of your friend's torso. Pull each hand, fingers pointing down, straight up from the table. Alternating hands, begin sliding one hand up just before the other is about to finish its pull so that there is no break between strokes. Begin pulling on the side of the hip just above the thigh and work your way up to the armpit, then back again. Move slowly, steadily, and just the width of one of your hands with each stroke.

When you are ready to massage the other side, keeping hand contact, walk to the other side of the table and repeat the Side Pulls on your friend's other side.

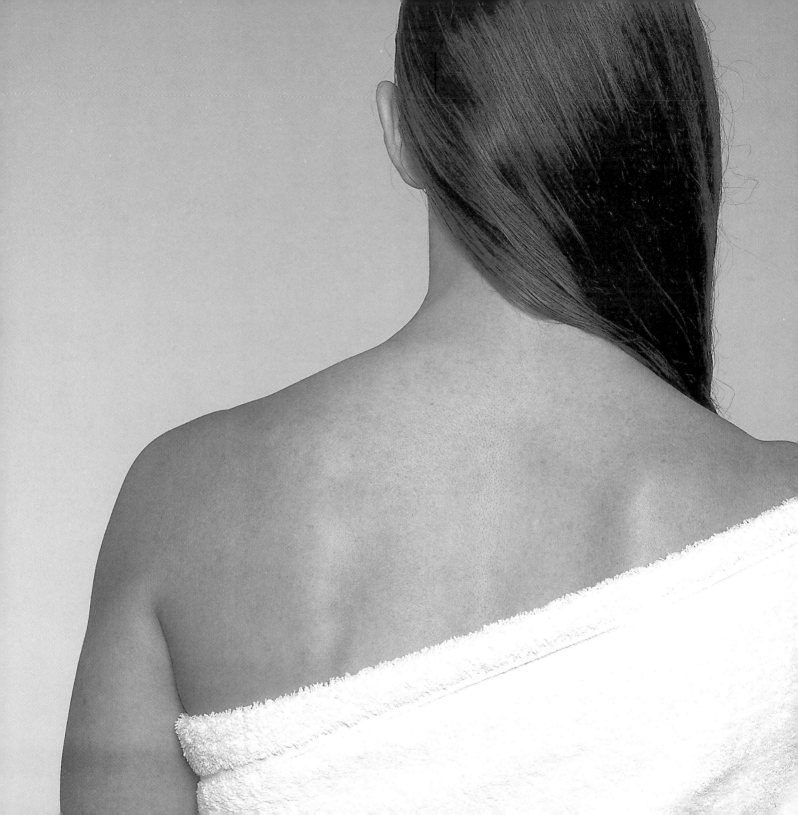

Shoulder Blade Exploration

If you want to work on an often tense area of the midback, have your friend roll over and do this stroke.

To reach the muscles threading under the shoulder blades, you will need to raise one of the blades a bit. Standing at your friend's right side, take his or her right hand and position it palm up on the middle of the back. Now lift the shoulder just off the table and slide your right forearm, underside up, under the shoulder so that it can rest at the crook of your elbow. With your right hand, steady your friend's forearm near his elbow. The key muscles to massage run in the furrow around the top, the side nearest the spine, and the bottom of the now raised blade. Glide the fingertips of your left hand several times firmly back and forth along all three sides.

Next make small circles with your fingertips, covering all three sides several times. Then shape your left hand as if it were a claw and press firmly on the blade itself, moving the skin in small circles slightly over the blade. To release the arm, slide your hand down the length of the arm and place it back on the table. Gently move your forearm from under his shoulder.

Repeat this sequence on the other shoulder blade standing by your friend's other side.

Waist Circle

After the Shoulder Blade Exploration, have your friend roll over onto his or her back again: then do the Waist Circle. Slide both hands, palms up, one from one side and one from the other, under your friend's back at the waistline. Bring your fingertips to either side of the spine.

With the backs of your hands against the table, press the fingertips of both hands up as hard as you can on either side of the spine. You may even raise the middle of your friend's body up a bit. Hold for several seconds and release. Now slide your hands, still pressing but more lightly, out from under the back and onto the center of the stomach. Articulate the waistline as you go.

Chest Palms

Stand above your friend's head. Place both your palms on your friend's shoulder pockets. Rest them there a while. Imagine you can send light and warmth down your arms to fill the chest.

Massage Doubled

A massage is an act of caring at any time. When two people massage someone, this can double the gift. That "extra" person joining the massage gives the feeling of extra luxury. It is also fun to do, offering new ways to experiment and invent strokes.

If the people giving the massage are a couple, they can expand their nonverbal communication skills and have the satisfaction of doing something together for someone else. Compassion is not always a solitary act. When you care for someone together, you become closer yourselves.

Being massaged by two people is either double pleasure or double trouble. It has to be done in a sensitive, synchronized way, or it feels very confusing and irritating. Each of the two giving the massage needs to tune in as fully to their massage partner as to the person receiving it.

As in water ballet, the key is to match your movement, your pressure, and your rhythm as closely as possible. Try to keep your movements exactly parallel, neither of you leading, neither following. Working on different areas, you won't be able to match strokes, but you can match rhythm and pace.

Begin by each holding one of your friend's feet with one hand under the sole and the other on the top. Imagine that your breath can travel down your arms and into your hands as they rest in place for a moment. Now spread massage oil on the leg or the foot that you were holding.

Remember to move up the legs at the same pace, crossing each body part and dividing your hands at junctures at exactly the same moment. When one of you is working solo on a small area—the head, for example—the other can go to work on the feet or the hands to maintain a sense of balance.

Double Main Stroke

Each of you stands by one leg. Slide both hands up the back of the leg. Your hands point in opposite directions and stay together. At the top of the leg, continue over the hip and buttock and up one side of the back muscles. Separate the hands and pivot them. When you reach the shoulder blade on your side of the body, draw the hands, heels first, down the side of the back and the leg and all the way back to the ankle. Repeat several times without pausing between strokes.

> *Aristotle asserted that the heart, not the brain, was the seat of intelligence and sensation.*

The Huge Hand

Secure four hands together by sliding your fingers in between each other, as though you were sliding two combs teeth to teeth. This will create a huge surface that the two of you can glide in any direction.

You are standing on opposite sides of the back facing each other and leaning into your interlocked hands. Begin to sculpt the contours of the back with your new huge massage hand. Without separating your fingers, draw the Huge Hand down one side of the ribs, then up onto the center of the back and down the other. Continue sculpting the back contours.

Two Bears Walking

Each of you leans across the table and presses one palm down on the top of the far side of your friend's back, just beyond the spine. Angle as much of your weight into the heel of your hand as you can. Now press your other hand beside the first just below it on the back. Next cross your first hand over and press it immediately below the second. Continue pressing with one hand just as you release with the other. "Bear walk" down the side of the back, over the buttocks, and down the legs. One exception to deep pressure is to touch very lightly on the backs of the knees. "Bear Walk" up the body to the shoulders.

Overlapping Palms

While your friend is lying on her stomach or back, stand on opposite sides of the table. Reaching across to touch the side of your friend's torso farthest from you, alternate your arms between your partner's arms. Keep all four arms close together.

Now begin the Overlapping Palms stroke in unison. Each of you slides one palm up his or her side of the torso. Just as your hand leaves the body, start your other palm stroking up the side. Establish an even rhythm for all four hands and work from the waist to the armpit and back down to the hips.

Main Stroke

Repeat the first stroke of the massage several times.

Full Feathers and Claws

Using only the tips of the fingers of both hands, and touching as lightly as you can on the surface of the skin, administer a series of feather-light strokes down the neck, back, and legs, all the way to the feet. You can alternate using your fingertips with using your nails for a subtle change of texture. Finish with feather-light stroking with your fingertips.

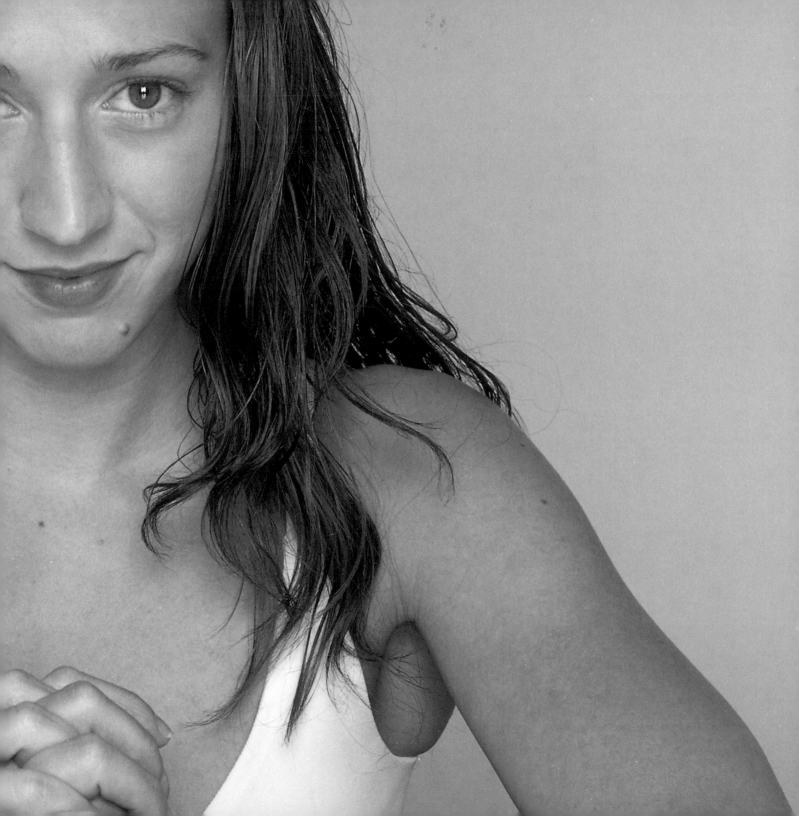

Throat Plexus

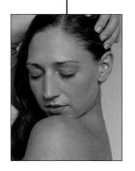

The Throat Plexus is centered in the throat area and includes the base of the neck, the upper shoulders, the arms and hands, and the nerves and body chemicals that guide feelings through this area.

Spirit Spa:
Meditation on Willpower

- Psychological associations: ability to make decisions and create.

- Massage for hands, arms, shoulders, and base of neck.

- The healing element is ether. The symbolic color is blue.

- Healing scents and oils include East Indian sandalwood, spearmint, Canadian balsam, sweet orange, frankincense, and Roman chamomile.

My Throat, My Communication

Psychologically, the throat is the center of communication. The mouth is viewed as a kind of doorway through which our inner thoughts can cross to the outside world. Because speech comes out of our mouths, the mouth is symbolic of creating something from nothing. In many spiritual traditions, a word is thought to have been the first creation of God and therefore is symbolic of original divine creation. Thus, singing is considered a holy part of religious ritual.

The arm and hand are linked to the throat in their shared symbolism of external creation. Arms and hands make things, build things, harm or shield things. Because of the hand's role in work and creation, it is a symbol of action in the exterior world. A closed fist symbolizes defense or attacks. An open hand symbolizes creation, receptivity, and healing.

White Birch and Orange Blossom Aromatherapy

White birch has a bracing scent that encourages calm confidence. Orange blossom scent encourages emotional balance.

Meditation on Willpower

You may light a candle or heat an essential oil incense with the scent of one of the healing herbs for this area.

Sit on a mat on the floor with a small pillow under your tailbone for support. Relax your hands, palms up, on your knees. Circle each thumb to its forefinger. Repeat the following breathing sequence ten times to relax the throat area, and clear the lungs by lengthening the exhalation.

With your mouth closed, slightly close the glottis at the back of your throat as you inhale through your nose, so that you produce a light snoring sound.

With your mouth still closed, exhale slowly through your nose as you produce a low humming sound in your throat. You may imagine that your throat area is bathed in a pale blue light.

As you meditate, you may focus on aspects of your emotional issues related to the powers of this body area. Silently ask yourself a question. Allow answers to surface, be noted, and dissolve.

Do I follow through on my plans? Why?
Do I believe in my dreams and
*   aspirations enough to live them?*
What is the source of my faith
*   in my own strength?*
What nourishes my sense of strength?
What undermines my resolutions?
Am I comfortable making choices and
*   acting on them?*
Do I have bad habits and addictions?
What are my excuses to myself for
*   continuing them?*
What helps me move beyond
*   self-destructive habits?*
How can I strengthen my willpower
*   today?*

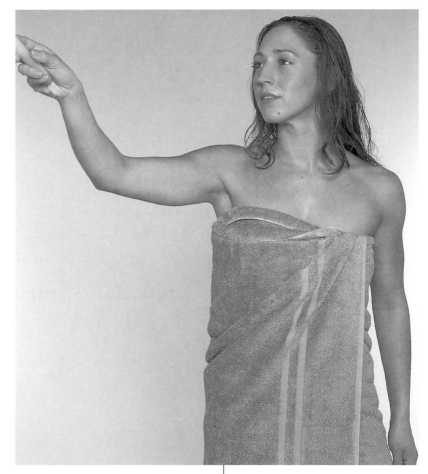

Kundalini

The spine contains one of the body's most powerful energy sources. In yoga, this energy is called *kundalini*. The current begins at the base of the spine and travels up through the top of the spinal cord into the brain. It is thought that when this current reaches the brain, it stimulates mental clarity and power. The more you can charge this current through visualization, breathing, and exercise, the more profound your mental awakening will be. As each energy center along the spine is stimulated, spiritual understanding opens in the person. The deepest yoga understanding is a realization of our unity with everyone and everything.

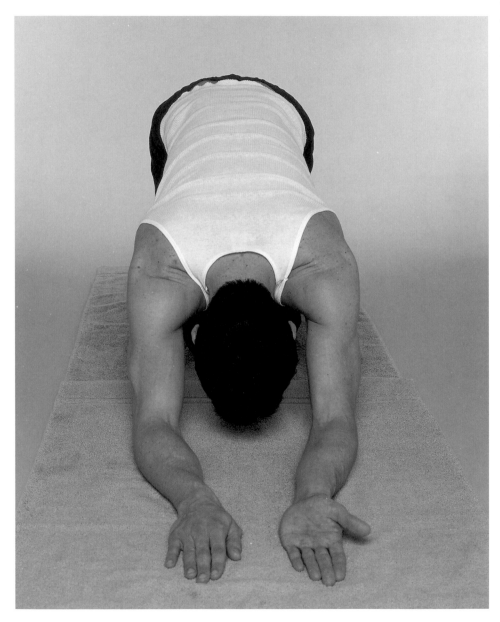

Breath of Fire

The Breath of Fire is a yoga technique involving a quick, forceful exhalation that pulls in your midriff, followed by deep inhalation that presses out the abdomen. Pump your lungs faster than during most other yoga breathing, use muscles more forcefully, and apply prana locks at different points. These techniques increase the effects of the breathing on your circulatory system and your mental functions.

Breath of Fire can be used simply to improve circulation and revive waning energy. Or it can be used in special sequences to raise the body's kundalini energy up the spine to stimulate higher spiritual centers in your head. This increases your physical strength as well as your emotional sense of confidence and willpower.

When you do the breathing exercise, the nerves send strong currents up the spine. It begins with a warmth in the lower back. This sensation can move up the spine and revitalize you. This is an advanced process, but a simple version of the Breath of Fire can be done effectively.

1 Sit upright. Breathe through your nose. As you inhale, puff your abdomen out. As you exhale, contract the abdominal muscles sharply inward. Increase the pace as you go. The breathing becomes deep, rapid, and forceful.

2 Quite the opposite of most yoga breathing patterns, the exhalation is short and hard, while the inhalation is slower and longer in a one-to-four ratio. Focus your attention on the solar plexus at your diaphragm as you exhale and on your throat chakra as you inhale.

3 After about forty breaths, inhale and hold your breath for a count of forty. When you exhale, do so slowly and evenly. Then begin the rapid Breath of Fire. After several minutes of this pattern, relax, breathe normally, and observe your response.

Beads Meditation

Many spiritual traditions use counting strings of beads, popularly know as worry beads, during meditation to calm anxiety and clear the mind of stress.

Use a string of 108 round beads plus one odd-shaped larger marker bead. Sit in a comfortable meditation position. Hold the marker bead in one hand resting on your lap. Close your eyes and say a sacred word, such as Aum, God, Love, or One, each time you touch a new bead. Touch each separate bead around the whole necklace, allowing anxious feelings and thoughts to pass out of your mind as you focus on the spiritual words.

Body Spa:
Shoulder, Arm, and Hand Massage

Orange Blossom Massage Oil

- 1 cup pure almond oil
- 4 drops orange blossom essential oil

Combine the oils in a plastic squeeze bottle. Orange blossom oil is soothing to the skin. The scent is calming and helps balance emotional tension and improve confidence.

Roman Chamomile and White Birch Hand Lotion

- $\frac{1}{4}$ cup olive oil
- 2 drops white birch essential oil
- 2 drops Roman chamomile essential oil

Combine the oils in a glass or ceramic bottle with a pump top. Roman chamomile is especially soothing and restorative to the skin. White birch helps relieve a variety of skin disorders, including eczema and psoriasis, as well as soothes arthritis and muscle pain. Olive oil maintains moisture balance and enriches the skin with vitamins.

Arm and Hand Glide

Position your friend's right arm at his or her side with the palm turned down. Smooth oil on the arm and shoulder.

Placing both your palms down across your friend's wrist, curve them so that they cover the top and the sides of the wrist. Start with your hands side by side, thumbs touching. Press firmly as you slide both hands together up the arm. When you reach the top of the arm, glide the left hand over the top of the shoulder and move the right down the inside of the arm just below the armpit.

Now, pressing lightly, glide both hands back down the arm, with your left hand on the outside and your right on the inside. When you reach the wrist you have two options. One is to slide your left hand onto the top of the wrist so that both hands resume positions to begin the same stroke again. The other is to slide both hands down your friend's hand and off his or her fingertips. Your right hand moves along the top of the hand and your left hand is underneath. Immediately after you leave the fingertips, move your hands into the starting position for another stroke so that your friend senses very little break in contact or pace.

Palm Fist*

Rest your friend's hand, palm up, in the palm of your left hand. Make a fist with your right hand. Pressing firmly, move your knuckles in small circles over the delicate valleys and ridges of the palm. Cover the entire palm.

All Thumbs on the Hand

Use both thumbs moving away from each other in overlapping strokes. Rhythmically and thoroughly massage the back of the hand with the tips of your thumbs, even venturing an inch or two onto the wrist. Then turn the hand over and, resting it on your fingers, use your thumbs to massage the palm and inside of the wrist thoroughly.

Hand Definition*

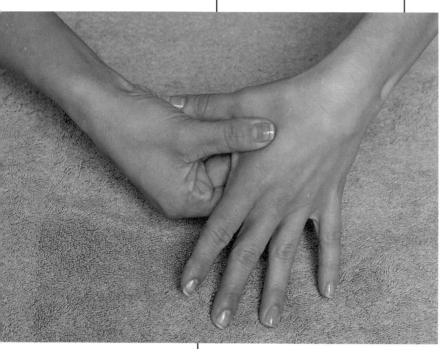

The small cords on the top of the hand, just under the surface of the skin, that run from the base of the wrist to the first knuckle of each finger are the metacarpal bones. To see them clearly, raise them by stretching all your fingers as far out and back as you can. Think of the metacarpals as ridges and the spaces between them as valleys in order to visualize this massage stroke.

Hold your friend's lightly oiled hand, palm down, in your left hand. Using firm pressure, slowly glide the tip of your thumb down each valley in turn, all the way from the base of the wrist to the small web of skin between each successive pair of fingers. It is usually most comfortable to use your right thumb to massage the two valleys nearest the right side of the hand and your left thumb on the valleys nearest the left.

When your thumb reaches the little flap of skin between two fingers, press the underside with the tip of your forefinger as your thumb presses from above, treating the area to a gentle pinch as your fingers slide off it. This flourish adds a sense of completion to the Hand Definition.

A person's fingerprint pattern is essentially unique. Statistical probability for two persons with duplicate fingerprints occurring is once every four billion years.

Draining the Arm

Raise your friend's forearm so that it is resting against your waist and upright with the elbow on the table. Circle the wrist with the thumbs and forefingers of both your hands; face your hands away from you so that your palms are tilted up as you hold the wrist. Your thumbs are touching each other and resting against the inside of the wrist. Your hand position is similar to the basic grip of a golf club.

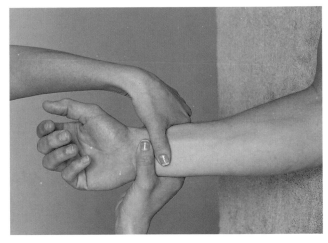

Squeeze lightly with your thumbs and fingers as you slide both hands slowly down the forearm as if you were draining it of excess moisture. Reach the crook of the elbow, then glide both hands back up the forearm again, keeping your thumbs and forefingers in contact with the skin but applying no pressure. Repeat the sequence several times.

You use pressure sliding down the forearm toward the elbow but not coming up, because the veins, which lie closer to the skin's surface than the arteries, are more affected by external pressure. Traditionally in massage you focus stroke pressure toward the heart to offer assistance to the voyage of the blood circulating through the veins toward the heart. A number of the other strokes, such as the leg strokes, also apply this pressure sequence. But on many strokes this sequence does not matter greatly, and the massage feels good either way. When you have given and received a great number of massages, you will develop a clear sense of when to deepen and when to lighten pressure. Studying anatomy charts also helps guide you.

Waitresses who touch their customers on the shoulder or hand as they return change generally receive larger tips than those who did not.

Thumb Glide on the Forearm

Hold your friend's forearm in the same upright position as you used for the draining stroke. With the fingers of both of your hands against the back of your friend's wrist for leverage, massage the inside of the wrist with the balls of your thumbs. Alternate each downward stroke out toward one or the other side of the wrist. Stroke downward until you have massaged all the muscles along the inside of the forearm.

Elbow Circles*

This technique is a treat for the often neglected elbow. With your friend's forearm still upright, make a loose fist with one hand and use it to gently massage the tender inside area—the crook—of the elbow with your knuckles. Next, lifting the upper arm slightly off the table with one hand, use the tips of the thumb and fingers of your other hand to massage the bony outside of the elbow. Massage in tiny circles over the entire elbow.

Neck Main Stroke

Position the palms of your hands, fingers pointing toward the shoulders, on your friend's shoulders. Slowly pivot the heels of your hands on top of your friend's shoulder to slide your fingers down the side of each shoulder, then under the shoulder, and down the back. Move your hands across the top of the back toward the spine. Just before reaching the spine, pull your hands up onto the back of the neck.

Glide your fingertips up the back of the neck. As they near the hairline, angle your hands so that your fingers are pointing upward toward the chin. Applying lighter pressure, slide back down the side of the neck.

When you reach the crook of the neck, your hands glide across the top of the chest out to the shoulder. From there begin the same stroke again. Moving in a continuous motion, repeat the whole sequence several times.

Neck Circles

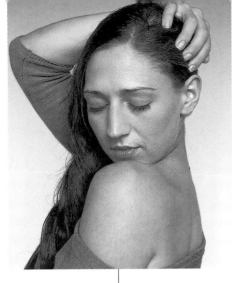

Tilt the head to the left to expose the muscles on the right side of the neck and shoulder. With the fingers of the right hand, make slow, firm circles about an inch wide against the back of the neck. Work from the base of the neck up to the hairline. Next, pressing more gently, make circles down the side of the neck, from below the ear down to the collarbone.

Trapezius Squeeze*

The upper portion of the trapezius reaches down your neck and across the top of your back and shoulders. These muscles form an area of high tension for most people. Constriction there often corresponds to conflicts over assertion. Popular body language defines "stiff-necked" people as inflexible, grumpy, uptight. You could probably measure a person's pent-up aggression by how high their shoulders rise during a tense situation. As a person releases tension, the muscles lengthen and the shoulders drop lower. These busy muscles need a lot of attention during a massage.

Standing at one end of the table behind your friend's head, use both hands and squeeze the trapezius muscles, with your thumbs on top and your forefingers underneath the shoulders. Maintain a rhythmic motion to massage these large muscles several times. Be sure you use plenty of oil so that your strokes slide over the skin.

Now, pressing your thumbs on top of the trapezius muscles, make small circles all over the area, leaning in with your body weight. Make these small thumb circles all over the back of the neck and shoulders and down the lower half of the trapezius muscles, between the shoulder blades.

Full Feathers

Using only the tips of the fingers of both hands and touching as lightly as you can on the surface of the skin, administer a series of feather-light strokes down the neck, arms, and legs, all the way to the feet.

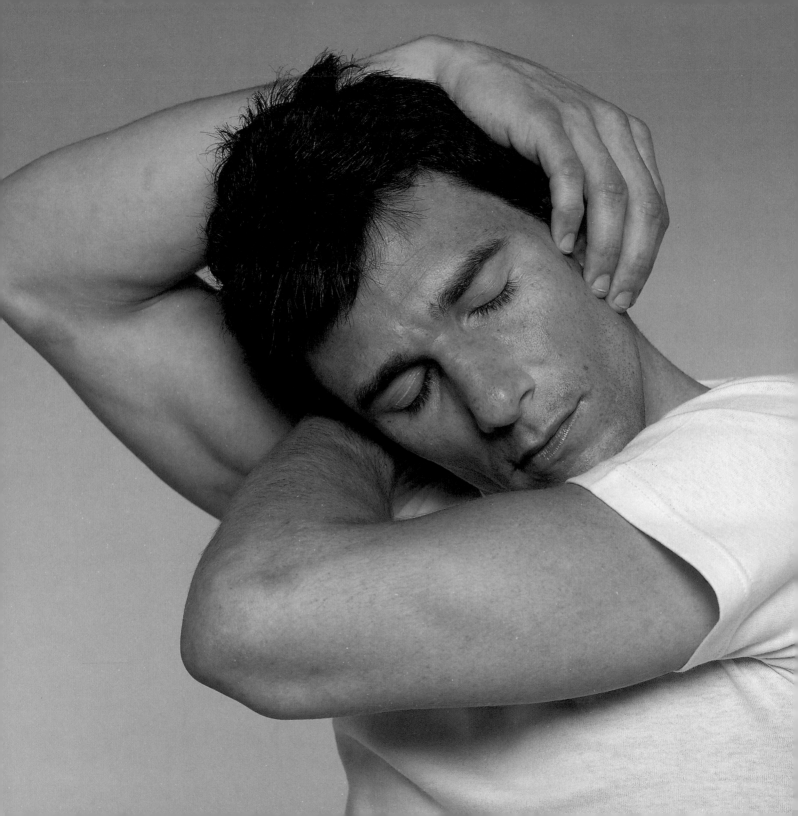

Forehead Plexus

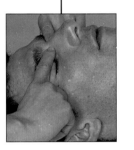

The Forehead Plexus is centered in the face, ears, and base of the skull, including the pituitary gland, the nervous system, and the medulla of the brain.

Spirit Spa:
Meditation on Honesty and Clarity

- Psychological associations: emotional and intelligence; ability to evaluate self and to perceive others.

- Massage for face and neck.

- The healing element is the mind. The symbolic color is yellow.

- Healing scents and oils include cardamom, vetiver, coriander, spearmint, lavender vera, and damask rose.

My Eyes, My Insight

Psychologically, the eyes are associated with clarity of perception, of others as well as of oneself. They are connected with light and thus are a symbol of receiving and sending out light, or intelligence and understanding. Since having two eyes is the human norm, possessing a third eye is a symbol of the superhuman or divine. Thus many religious paintings show an extra eye in the center of the forehead to represent divine understanding. Eyes painted on other body parts depict the use of that part for high spiritual purposes. The face is the symbol of how we show ourselves to the world and of our ability to look at challenges with courage and honesty. Being "two-faced" means being dishonest.

Cardamom and Sandalwood Aromatherapy

Add a few drops of cardamom oil to East Indian sandalwood oil for a heady meditation incense. Cardamom relieves nervous strain and mental fatigue. Indian sandalwood lifts depression and relieves insomnia and stress reactions. In Asia, sandalwood is a favorite building material for temples.

Spearmint Aromatherapy

Spearmint helps relieve sinusitis, headache, fatigue, and nervous strain. The oil is beneficial to the skin. The scent targets the head and sinus area.

Cucumber Eye Mask

Successful simplicity should not be ignored. Unadorned cucumber slices have been used to soothe tired eyes for centuries. Lie down and close your eyes. Place a round chilled cucumber slice on top of each eyelid. Relax a while.

Meditation on Honesty

You may light a candle or heat incense with one of the healing herb scents for this area. Sit in a comfortable lotus position on a mat on the floor. Place a small pillow under your tailbone. Relax your hands, palms up, on your knees. Circle each thumb to its forefinger.

Close your eyes. Turn your eyes up and focus them toward the space between the eyebrows. This is the location of the pituitary gland, or "Third Eye," which when stimulated increases intuition and clarity of thought. Directing your eye gaze at this point stimulates the olfactory nerves, optic nerves, and central nervous system. Start by holding this gaze for one to two minutes. Gradually increase to ten minutes, but no longer. Holding too long strains the eyes and nerves. However long you hold the gaze, spend the same amount of time after relaxing the eyes in a level gaze position.

Each time you meditate, you may focus on one aspect of your emotional issues related to the powers of this body area. Allow answers to the questions to surface and then dissolve.

How honest am I with myself when I evaluate
   my actions and motives?
How truthful am I with others?
How open am I to new information and ideas of others?
Which of my attitudes form barriers to perceiving
   others accurately and to communicating honestly?
Which of my attitudes nourish truthfulness?
What can I do today to live more honestly?

As you meditate, imagine that a warm, golden light is glowing at the spot in the center of your forehead between your eyes.

Watching the Clock

This exercise strengthens the eye muscles and improves the eyesight. Start with brief sessions and gradually increase the length.

1 Sit in a comfortable meditation pose with spine erect. Close your eyes.

2 Imagine your face has a clock painted on it. Keeping your lids closed, look up as far as you can at a spot in the center of your forehead where the number twelve would be on the clock. Hold this gaze for a count of five.

3 Shift your gaze a bit to the right, as though you are looking at the number one of the clock, about the middle of your right eyebrow. Hold this gaze for five seconds.

4 Shift your gaze to the far corner of your right eye, where the number two would be. Hold the gaze for about five seconds.

5 Continue around your face in a clockwise direction, stopping at each imaginary number until you reach twelve again.

6 Then reverse the process and gaze at each number in a counterclockwise sequence. Rest a moment with closed eyes, then open them slowly.

Mandala Meditation

Mandalas consist of circular geometric forms that suggest the concentric patterns making up all levels of life forms, from the cell to the solar system. A mandala is a blueprint of the architecture of the natural world. In Sanskrit, *mandala* means "center" and "circle." From the snowflake to the cyclone, natural systems rotate around a central energy point. The center of the mandala design symbolizes the mysterious, inexhaustible source of all creation.

Mandalas are usually very beautiful, and are designed primarily to stimulate spiritual awakening in us as we concentrate on the center and allow our perceptions to align with the concentric patterns. The psychologist Carl Jung used mandalas as therapeutic devices for calming his patients. Painting them and gazing at them are meditation rituals. A good book for pictures of mandalas is *Mandala* by Jose Arguelles, Chogyam Trungpa, and Miriam Arguelles.

Any balanced concentric form can function as a mandala. If color is added, more senses are awakened. You can study the symbolism of Asian colors or create your own symbolic cosmos. The male and female mandala symbolizes opposite elements in all of us that bring unity when balanced within ourselves and in the outside world.

Visualization

Visualization in the field of medicine refers to using healthy, positive images of your body to improve your physical and emotional conditions. Through this experience, your mind can revive your flagging energy and help heal sore or damaged muscles and tissue.

There are two steps in the process. For example, if you have a torn ligament, allow yourself to see an image in your mind's eye of the current state of that body part, imagining what the area looks like fragmented and inflamed. Next visualize how it should be. Looking at anatomy charts is useful. Throughout the day bring this healthy picture of your ligaments and muscles to mind to encourage healing.

This mental process of visualization is an ancient technique that shamans, yogis, witches, and other healers have used throughout history. Many Western medical doctors now use visualization effectively to help cancer patients and injured athletes. Visualization is useful for people who are in pain or are too tired or too sick to do other kinds of treatments or exercise. You can also try encouraging healing in other people by visualizing them healthy.

Visualization can be used as a form of practice that will improve your performance. Athletes often use visualization as part of their warm-up routines. Visualize yourself doing an exercise or sport before the event. Imagining something stimulates many of the same responses in your nerves and muscles as doing it. You can also use visualization throughout the day as a preventive technique by maintaining a healthy image of your body in top shape.

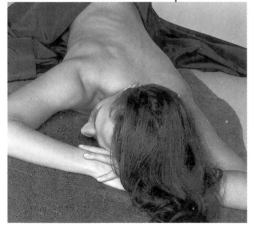

Mind Massage

Visualization can be used to explore an emotional or physical pain or tight muscle. Imagine you can shrink yourself and walk into your body to search and do internal maintenance. Don't preplan the story; simply try to let the events occur. They will.

Lie down, close your eyes, and relax your breathing. If you have a specific ache or pain you want to work on, locate it and then choose a natural body opening as your "entranceway." Imagine you can shrink yourself or someone else to about a half inch or smaller.

The journey in and out is just as important as the destination. Resist hurrying or missing any steps. You can talk out loud about what you are doing and how it feels to you. If you have a pain in your upper back you want to reach, you could enter through your mouth. Look around at the setting and describe it. "I am walking up to the mouth. I am crawling over the lips. As I let myself down inside, the surface becomes slippery. It's dark in here. I'm walking toward the back of the mouth on the teeth. They feel sharp and bumpy."

When you reach the back of the mouth, decide how to get down the throat and into the shoulder. "There's a deep hole here like a well. There's no way to get down except to jump, but I don't know where I'll land." You can decide to go on or try another way. "I think I'll just jump." Describe your descent, what you see, how you feel. Almost always, a surprise landing takes place; if not, pick something to grab onto to stop yourself when you feel you've fallen far enough.

When you land, decide how you're going to get to your sore muscle. You can swim through an artery or walk along a tendon. When you reach the sore muscle, look around. Describe what you see. Try to imagine a way you could massage the muscle by walking on it or squeezing it. Imagine you are doing this. Take your time.

When you have massaged to your satisfaction, begin your journey out of the body. Out again, imagine you can expand to your normal size and merge with your larger body. Take a moment to check how the previously sore muscle feels now. Often it feels greatly relaxed.

> *Approximately twenty million Americans suffer from chronic headaches and spend about three hundred million dollars a year on headache medicine.*

Body Spa:
Face Massage

Lavender and Vetiver Massage Oil

- 1 cup pure almond oil
- 1 teaspoon olive oil
- 1 teaspoon aloe vera oil
- 2 drops lavender vera oil
- 2 drops vetiver oil

Combine the oils in a plastic squeeze bottle. Almond oil lightly moisturizes. Olive and aloe vera oils enrich the skin with nutrients while balancing the acidity. Lavender oil and aroma relieve headache, insomnia, migraine, and nervous tension.

Damask Rose and Honey Face Mask

2   tablespoons honey
1½ teaspoons almond oil
4   drops damask rose essential oil

Combine the ingredients in a glass or ceramic bowl and apply to face and neck for about ten minutes. Rinse off with lukewarm water. Honey tightens the pores. Almond oil moisturizes. Rose oil is especially helpful in relieving puffiness, dry skin, and wrinkles.

Forehead Palms

Rest your palms, fingers facing each other, lightly against your friend's forehead. The heels of your hands rest down near the temples. Pause for several seconds. Center yourself and allow your friend to become accustomed to your touch.

Thumb Spreads

Place the sides of the tips of your thumbs next to each other in the middle of your friend's forehead near the hairline. Slide your thumbs away from each other. Cover the height of the forehead in a series of horizontal strokes that begin in the center and spread out toward the temples. End each stroke by tracing light circles on both temples. Then lift the thumbs off the face to resume their central position to start again.

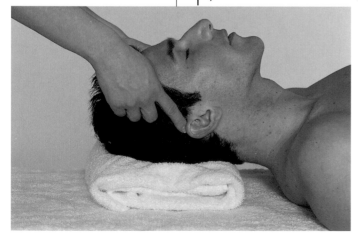

Finger Spreads*

Next massage under the cheekbones with the forefinger and the middle fingers of both hands. Place the tips of these fingers at the center of the face between the nose and the mouth. Cupping the fingers under the cheekbones, glide outward onto the cheeks, then end with a circle on the temples.

Now do several of the spreading strokes between the mouth and the tip of the chin. Start each stroke in the center and end on the temples.

To complete the face spreads, lightly press the center of the chin between the tips of the thumb and forefinger of each hand. Draw your fingers out to the edges of the jaw until you have almost reached the ears. Now glide the forefingers to a final circle on the temples.

> *Your circulatory system has two important jobs: transportation of materials and regulation of temperature.*

Eyelid Glide*

This gentle stroke is for the eyelids. Before starting, ask to make certain that your friend is not wearing contact lenses. Start just beside the nose and move outward. Move very slowly. Place one thumb or forefinger on each eyelid, pointing toward each other. Very lightly, run the balls of your thumb or forefinger straight across your friend's eyelids. Apply a minimum of pressure.

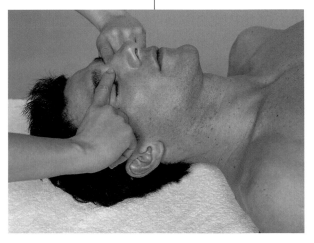

Ear Treats*

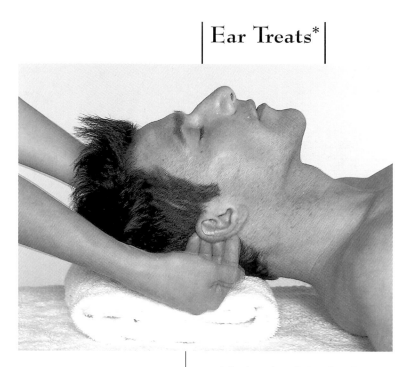

To start, work on one ear at a time. With practice you may prefer to massage both at once.

Hold the tips of your fingers together, forming a crescent, and several times slide them gently up and down the back of the ear where it connects with the rest of the head.

Place the length of your forefinger behind the ear and slide it several times up and down in the V formed by the topmost part of the ear and the skull.

Now lightly pinch the outer edge of the earlobe between your thumb and forefinger. Start next to the skull and work around, moving your thumb and forefinger a fraction of an inch between pinches.

With the tip of the forefinger, gently trace the curling valleys of the inside of the ear. Work from the outer edge toward the center, stopping just short of closing off the ear channel.

Chin Lifts*

Place the tips of the forefinger and the middle fingers of both hands at the center of the face between the mouth and the tip of the chin. Stroke outward onto the cheeks, then up to the temples, and end with a circle on the temples.

Next, lightly grasp the tip of the chin between the tips of the thumb and forefinger of each hand. Firmly pinch and slide your fingers over the edges of the jaw until you reach the ears. Then glide the forefingers and the middle fingers into a small circle on the temples.

Neck Loops

Begin with your palms resting on your friend's shoulders. With both hands moving at once, spread your palms away from each other and stroke down the sides of the shoulders. Then slide your hands under the shoulders and begin moving them toward each other on the upper back. Just before the hands would touch either side of the spine, pull them up onto the back of the neck. Slide your fingers up the neck to the base of the skull, without lifting the head off the table. Next slip your hands away from the body. Quickly return your palms to rest on top of the shoulders to begin the stroke again.

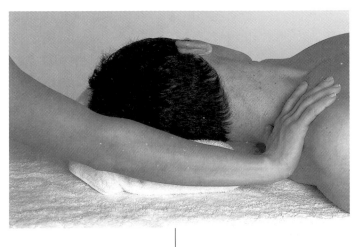

Eye Palms

Rest the heels of your hands on the top edges of the eye sockets. Each of your palms lightly cups over an eye socket. On either side of the nose, your fingers point toward the chin. Close your eyes and relax in this position for up to two minutes. Imagine you can send warmth and relaxation down your arms and into your hands, to relax the face and gradually the rest of your friend's body.

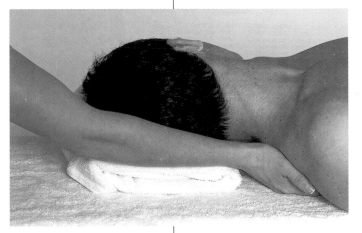

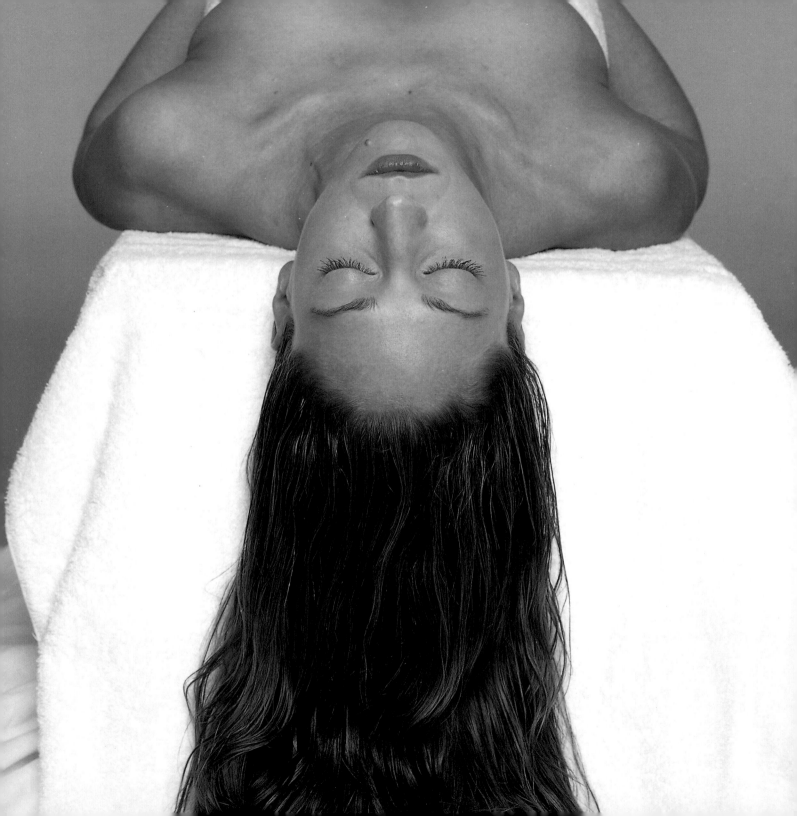

Cranial Plexus

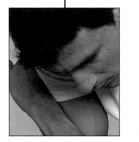

The Cranial Plexus is centered in the scalp and skull, including the pineal gland and the cerebral cortex.

Spirit Spa:
Meditation on Ethics and Perspective

- Psychological associations: values, courage, sense of spiritual responsibility to others.

- Massage for head and scalp.

- The healing element is spiritual consciousness. The symbolic color is white.

- Healing scents and oils include citronella, East Indian sandalwood, vetiver, patchouli, frankincense, lavender vera, and lemon balm.

My Head, My Spirituality

The top of the head is symbolic of a person's connection to higher spiritual powers. The skull is the symbolic crown of the body, representing higher powers directed upward. Since the head is a sphere, it is a symbol of oneness and centeredness. The skull inside the head is symbolic of the inseparable cycle of death and life. Hair generally symbolizes energy; thus, cutting it represents losing vitality. Spiritually, cutting your own hair symbolizes intentionally giving up physical power for spiritual insight. This is the meaning of the practice of monks shaving their heads.

Frankincense Meditation Incense

Used in spiritual rituals for thousands of years, frankincense slows the breathing when inhaled and thus is conducive to meditation and prayer. Applied to the skin, frankincense oil relieves dryness and scarring. The scent tends to have a calming effect and relieves anxiety and nervous tension.

Meditation on Ethics

You may heat an essential oil incense or light a candle with one of the healing scents for this chakra.

Sit in a comfortable lotus position on a mat on the floor. Place a small pillow under your tailbone. Relax your hands, palms up, on your knees. Touch the thumb of each hand to the forefinger.

Close your eyes. Focus your attention on the center of the top of your head. Imagine a small circle or sunburst of light there.

You may simply count your breaths as you imagine the light growing and expanding from your body into the air around you.

You may silently ask yourself some questions as you breathe, and allow the answers to appear and then disappear.

What do I value most in life?

What values are most important to me?

How far would I go to defend these values?

Do I hold myself accountable in all situations for living up to
*   these values? If I make exceptions, in what situations?*

Where did I learn these values?

Do I expect others to share my values?

How do I treat people who do not share my values?

Do I feel a sense of connection with a creative or divine
*   spirit in the universe?*

If not, would I like to feel this connection?

Whom do I know who exemplifies the spiritual values I admire?

What are the ways I know to increase my spiritual understanding
*   and action in the world?*

Lotus Meditation

The seventh energy center at the top of the head is often pictured in Indian literature as a lotus flower with a thousand petals. The six lower chakras are shown as flowers with only a few petals, but the highest energy center has many because all aspects of ourselves depend on our relationship to our highest energy, our spiritual power and openness. Try visualizing a beautiful lotus blossom with countless white petals opening to the sunlight. Imagine your heart and mind opening this gracefully to spiritual devotion and compassion.

Leonardo da Vinci's anatomical drawings offered medicine
the first precise picture of the brain's cavities.

Prana Seal

This posture helps sustain the benefits of your breathing exercises and unites opposing natural energies.

Sit in a meditation posture with your legs crossed. Perform your breathing exercises. Afterward, inhale through your nose as you wrap your arms behind your waist. Clasp your right wrist with your left hand.

Exhale as you lean your torso forward and relax your neck and forehead toward the floor. Rest in this position for as long as you feel comfortable.

The number of hairs a person has is set by the number of hair follicles, determined genetically before birth.

The Diamond Mantra

Aum Ah Hum Vajra Guru Padme Siddhi Hum
(ohm ahh hoom vahjrah goor oo pahdmay siddy hoom)

This Tibetan mantra builds your power to act with strength and compassion in a difficult world, to function with diamond clarity.

Aum: clear body
Ah: clear speech
Hum: clear mind
Vajra: diamond-sharp truth
Guru: wisdom
Padme: lotus symbolizing compassion
Siddhi: realization or blessing
Hum: may this come to pass (similar to Amen)

Chanting this sequence of words repeatedly for as long as is comfortable invokes the healing blessings of the divine spirit. You are requesting God to give you clarity in all your aspects so you can act with compassionate power in the world.

Body Spa:
Head Massage

Essential Oils for Hair and Scalp

Just before you step out for a sunny exercise session or into a warm bath, apply an herbal treatment to your scalp. It will soak in best when your pores widen in response to heat. Or you may put oil on your hair before your scalp massage. Later, when you wash your hair, use a cool or cold water final rinse to close the pores and leave your hair more shiny.

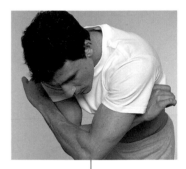

Lavender Scalp Conditioner

| 11 | drops essential lavender vera oil |
| $1/2$ | cup extra-virgin olive oil |

Once a week, apply this lavender oil to improve your hair's elasticity and alleviate scalp tension. Dampen your hair. Slightly warm the olive oil in a small saucepan. Remove from stove. Add lavender oil. Massage warm mixture into scalp. You may wear a plastic shower cap into the bath to increase the heat and absorption. Or go play in the sun with your lavender scented hair. Leave oil on for at least half an hour. Longer is better. Shampoo as usual.

Lemon and Apple Hair Rinse

$1/2$ cup organic apple cider vinegar
10 drops essential lemon balm oil
$1/2$ cup warm water

Mix in a jar and shake well in order to disperse the lemon balm oil before applying. After shampooing, allow hair to dry a bit, but leave damp. Massage this mixture into hair and scalp to remove soap and chemical film and to add shine.

Vetiver and Maple Hair Syrup

6 drops vetiver essential oil
$1/4$ to $1/2$ cup pure maple syrup, depending on hair volume

Stir to mix. Massage into damp hair and scalp. You may leave a light application on in the sunlight, or cover with a shower cap for indoor heat, for half an hour. Rinse, then shampoo as usual. The maple syrup adds moisture and shine to your hair. The vetiver is calming to muscles and mood.

Palming the Forehead

Rest your palms lightly against your friend's forehead for a few moments. The heels of your hands cover the forehead and the fingers curve down the temples. Pausing for several seconds allows you to center yourself and your friend to grow accustomed to your touch.

Eye Socket Points*

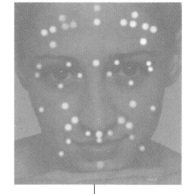

Press firmly with the tips of both forefingers against the bony rims of the two eye sockets, just inside where they meet the nose. Hold this deep pressure steadily for a count of two. Then slowly lift your forefingers and place them about a third of an inch farther along the upper half of each rim. Press down again. This steady pressure is good for the sinuses.

Continue moving to pressure points about a third of an inch apart until you have reached the outermost point, farthest from the nose, of each eye socket. Next return to the point nearest the nose and massage the length of the lower half of the eye rim in the same fashion.

Cheekbone Points*

Position the tips of the first three fingers of each hand just to either side of the nose and just below the rim of the cheekbone where it meets the nose. Press in firmly. Glide the tips of your fingers around the lower crescent edges of the cheekbones toward the ears. Then slide them back up to the temples to make a light circle there. Because this cheek and jaw area is a center for tension in the face, a little extra focus here goes a long way toward relaxation.

Scalp Rub*

Lift the head slightly with your left hand and turn it to the left. Holding your right hand in the taut shape of a claw, rub the scalp on the right side of the head with your fingertips. Pressing hard, move your hand in small circles. Do not loosely slide your fingertips across the surface of the skin. Press hard enough that you move the skin itself over the bone. Work in wide rows up and down the head so that you cover the whole right side of the scalp. Now repeat these circles on the other side of the skull.

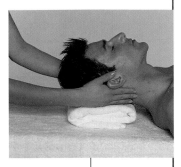

Craniosacral Pulse Rest

At the end of your Scalp Rub, find the bony ridge, or occipital ridge, on the back of the head where the skull meets the neck. Just above this ridge is a slight depression. Position your hands, palms up, on either side of the neck. Bend the first three fingers of each hand so that they press into the indention in the skull above and to either side of the center. This should lift the skull very slightly off the table so that the weight of the head now rests fully on your fingertips. Hold this position as long as you comfortably can. Allow your friend to relax his or her neck muscles more and more to give the weight over to you. Slight pressure on these spots helps still the craniosacral pulse, the rhythmic movement of the cerebrospinal fluid, to help relax and revive the whole body.

Head Turns

Position your hands securely under the back of your friend's head, holding up the head. Gently lift it a little and turn it slowly to the left. The head should now rest easily in your left hand. If you sense resistance or that your friend is trying to help, ask him to relax his neck muscles and let you do the work of holding up the head. Turn the head back to center. Gently raise and lower the head a few inches. Try the turn to the right now.

Twelve pairs of cranial nerves control your head and its sense organs, as well as some autonomic reactions.

Head Lift

Position both hands securely under your friend's head so that the skull is resting in your palms. Moving very slowly and evenly, lift the head as far forward as it will go.

Whenever you feel resistance, stop for a moment at that point. Then very gently nudge the head about an inch farther forward. If a gentle push isn't enough, then don't push at all. As you lower the head, move very slowly. Lightly return your friend's head to the table.

Head and Abdomen Centering

Stand to your friend's right as she is lying on his or her back. Rest the palm of your left hand lightly on his or her forehead. Place your right palm lightly on the abdomen just below the navel. Close your eyes. Relax your breathing. Allow a pause at the end of your exhalation before you breathe in again in order to allow your body to choose its own rhythm. Imagine that you can send your breath (or warmth or circulation or light) down your arms as you exhale.

Feel the increased heat in your palms. Now imagine you can send warmth and light from your hands into your friend's body. Your hands are placed to direct energy up the spine in order to strengthen the natural energy flow through the chakras, starting in the pelvis and spiraling up the spine to the head. The right hand has a positive charge flowing toward the left, which has a negative charge that attracts the positive. Thus you are directing energy to move up from the abdomen to be received in the head. Imagine that each chakra area starts to glow as the energy progresses up the body, until all the chakras are lit.

The chakras are like little moons, suns, or stars, whose light and warmth are increased by your attention. This light and warmth will circulate back to you through your arms. Because you and your friend have exchanged an act of caring and kindness, both of you have renewed your bodies and spirits. The energy from this simple act will spread out to grace the rest of the world with a little more warmth and light.

Chapter Index

SECTION TWO: SEVEN CENTERS OF HEALTH

Ch. 1: Pelvic Plexus

Spirit Spa

Body Spa

Ch. 2: Belly Plexus

Ch. 3: Solar Plexus

Spirit Spa

Body Spa

Ch. 4: Cardiac Plexus

Ch. 5: Throat Plexus

Spirit Spa

Body Spa

Ch. 6: Forehead Plexus

Spirit Spa

Ch. 7: Cranial Plexus

Spirit Spa

Self-Massage Strokes

Pelvic Plexus
Zone Therapy
Ankle Inside Point
Sole Revival
Knee Palms
Acupressure Tendon Revival
Leg Feathers

Belly Plexus
Acupressure Stomach Balance
Pelvis Pressure Points

Solar Plexus
Collarbone Outline

Cardiac Plexus
Collarbone Outline

Throat Plexus
Palm Fist
Hand Definition
Elbow Circles
Trapezius Squeeze

Forehead Plexus
Finger Spreads
Eyelid Glide
Ear Treats
Chin Lifts

Cranial Plexus
Eye Socket Points
Cheekbone Points
Scalp Rub

Further Reading

Arguelles, Jose, Chogyam Trungpa, and Miriam Arguelles. *Mandala*. Boston: Shambhala Publishing, 1995.

Capra, Fritjov. *The Tao of Physics: An Exploration of the Parallels Between Modern Physics and Eastern Mysticism*. Boston: Shambhala Publishing, 1991.

Chopra, Deepak, M.D. *Ageless Body, Timeless Mind: The Quantum Alternative to Growing Old*. New York: Three Rivers Press, 1998.

Downing, George. *The Massage Book*. New York: Random House, 1998.

Hanh, Thich Nhat. *The Blooming of a Lotus: Guided Meditation Exercises for Healing and Transformation*. Boston: Beacon Press, 1993.
————. *Going Home: Jesus and Buddha as Brothers*. New York: Riverhead Books, 1999.

The Dalai Lama. *The Path to Tranquility*. New York: Viking, 1999.
————. *Ethics for the New Millennium*. New York: Riverhead Books, 2000.

Manaka, Yoshio. *The Layman's Guide to Acupuncture*. New York: Weatherhill, 1975.

Myss, Caroline, Ph.D. *Anatomy of the Spirit: The Seven Stages of Power and Healing*. New York: Three Rivers Press, 1996.

Pert, Candace, Ph.D. *Molecules of Emotion: Why You Feel the Way You Feel*. New York: Simon & Schuster, 1999.

Rush, Anne Kent. *The Back Rub Book: How to Give and Receive Great Back Rubs*. New York: Vintage, 1989.
————. *Bodywork Basics: A Guide to the Powers and Pleasures of Your Body*. New York: Dell, 2000.
————. *Romantic Massage: Ten Unforgettable Massages for Special Occasions*. New York: Avon, 1991.

Suzuki, Shunryn. *Zen Mind, Beginner's Mind*. New York: Weatherhill, 1988.

Vishnudevananda, Swami. *The Complete Illustrated Book of Yoga*. New York: Crown, 1995.

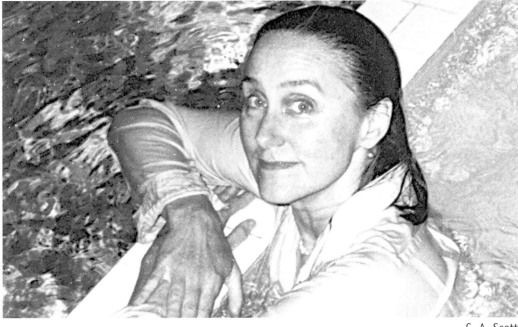

C. A. Scott

Anne Kent Rush has written more than a dozen books on preventive health care, including the Dell trilogy, *The Modern Book of Massage*, *The Modern Book of Yoga,* and *The Modern Book of Stretching*. In addition, she cocreated the pioneering two-million-selling manual, *The Massage Book* by George Downing, as well as authored the best-selling titles *Getting Clear: Bodywork for Women*, *The Back Rub Book*, and *Romantic Massage*. Rush has served on the teaching staff at Esalen Institute in San Francisco and Big Sur, where she helped found the women's studies program. After conducting a ten-year private practice in body therapy in California, Rush moved to the shores of the Gulf of Mexico, where she continues her work in preventive health care.